THE POWER OF
BREATHING

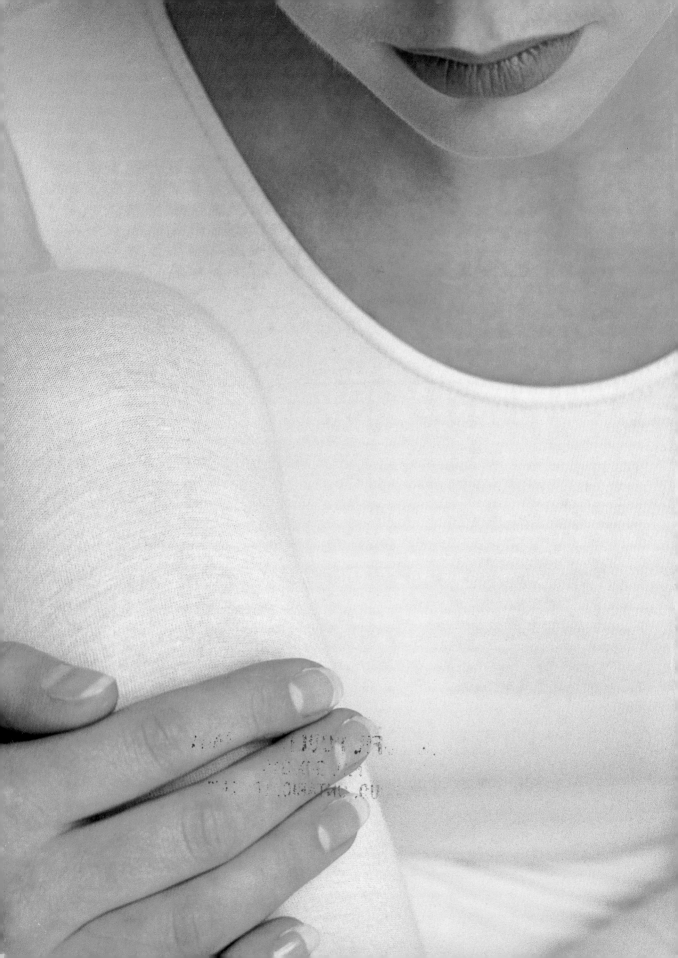

THE POWER OF
BREATHING

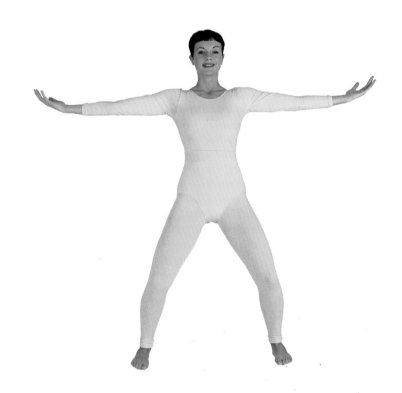

UTE GERZABEK

MARSHALL PUBLISHING • LONDON

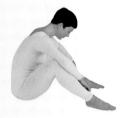

A Marshall Edition
Edited and designed by
Marshall Editions Ltd
The Orangery
161 New Bond Street
London W1Y 9PA

First published in the UK in 1999 by
Marshall Publishing Ltd

ISBN 1-84028-251-7
9 8 7 6 5 4 3 2 1

Originated in Singapore by PICA Colour Separation Pte
Printed in Portugal by Printer Portuguesa

Project Editor Wendy James
Designers Hugh Schermuly
            Joanna Stawarz
Managing Editor Anne Yelland
Managing Art Editor Patrick Carpenter
Copy Editor Lindsay McTeague
DTP Editor Lesley Gilbert
Editorial Coordinator Rebecca Clunes
Index Laura Hicks
Editorial Director Ellen Dupont
Art Director Sean Keogh
Production Nikki Ingram, Sarah Hinks

Contents

Foreword   6

Introduction
You are your best teacher   8

Part 1
A guide to breathing freely   10

What you can achieve from this book   12
   Breathing awareness   13
The way we breathe   14
The effects of breath training   16
Effective exercising   18
The basics for all exercises   20
About the exercises   32
   Establishing a routine   33

Part 2
The exercises   34

Discover the power of breathing   36
   Warming up   37
   Become aware of your breathing   38
Be at home with yourself   42
   The sitting bones   42
   Ribs and diaphragm   46
The Pendulum – to stretch and straighten the body   48
   Getting into the swing   48
   Rhythm and movement   52
   Regaining control   54
The Cradle – strengthening leg, stomach and back muscles   56
   Rocking and rolling   56
The Cat – encouraging flexibility   62
   Shoulder lift: breathing areas 3 and 7   62
   Stretch and strengthen   63
   Side twist: breathing area 2   66
   A longer stretch: breathing areas 1 and 3   66

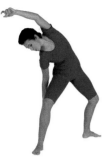

The Cloud – increasing the use of the diaphragm | 70
   Expand and accumulate: breathing areas 3 and 4 | 72
The Root – improving your level of fitness | 76
   Strength and stability: breathing areas 1 and 2 | 76
The Flower — opening breathing areas 3 and 7 | 84
   Extend and stretch: breathing areas 3 and 7 | 84
The Ball – vitalizing your breathing reflex | 92
   Feel your breathing | 93
   Breathe and bounce | 94
   Tense and stretch | 96
   Tense and bounce | 98
The Wave – stimulating all the breathing areas and circulation | 100
   Rhythm and rolling | 100
   Extend your breathing | 102
   Rolling out tension | 104

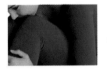

Part 3
Breathing through the day   **106**

Everyday well-being | 108
   Say good morning to your system | 109
   Moving into the day | 110
   Energy boost | 110
   Fuelling yourself | 111
   Last-minute tension busters | 112
Get into the day's rhythm | 113
   Dangers of holding the breath | 113
Tactics to overcome shallow breathing | 115
Letting go now and then | 118
Self-help guide to everyday ailments and conditions | 120
   Chronic conditions | 124
   Do's and don'ts | 124
Posture and breathing | 125

Index | 126
Acknowledgments | 128

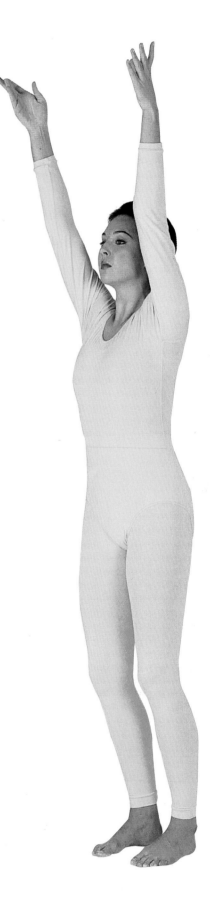

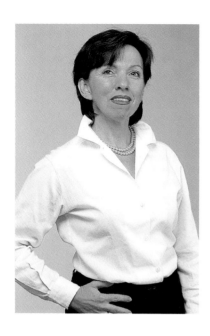

Foreword

The idea to write a book about my method of breath training came from my students, those I have taught at the University of Music and Performing Arts in Vienna or privately, and those who have attended my numerous seminars. They repeatedly asked if there was a book on the subject to complement my training. And here it is.

I developed this extensive training programme from my experiences as a professional singer and teacher. It includes some techniques you may recognize – such as practices developed by Feldenkreis, Middendorf and Wolf, Alexander and Eutonie, and various Eastern methods which certainly have had some influence on me. But the aim of my programme is continuity, to encourage you to practise breathing in the way you would learn an instrument, step by step.

By following the range of exercises, by repeating the sequences within them again and again, you will see progress and change in yourself. Once you have mastered the techniques you will be able to adjust your breathing to any situation you meet in your daily life.

Becoming aware of your breathing, sensing and experiencing it, is subtle work but it will soon reveal much about your body that may be new to you. Conscious breathing opens up important dimensions. With its power and energy, breath is a source of vitality. You are missing out if you watch idly while energy flows in when you inhale and escapes again when you exhale. Conscious breathing gives you the opportunity to take part actively in this process. And you can turn this power to good use.

The specially designed exercises will affect your whole being, body and mind. Many things will become easier to do. Aches and pains will be less severe, and may even disappear. You will become more confident and, last but not least, your posture will improve. This makes your blood circulation more efficient and you will feel more stimulated, physically and mentally. Through training your breathing, you will find a renewed vigour and zest for life.

Introduction

You are your best teacher

Your breathing is as individual as you are. It is essential to life, and making you conscious of every aspect of it – its form, dimension and rhythm – is the purpose of this book. Once you know more about these factors you will discover just how much power you have to improve your overall health and general well-being. How is this done? It is achieved through training your breathing. And such training benefits everyone, not just those who use their voices professionally for speaking or singing.

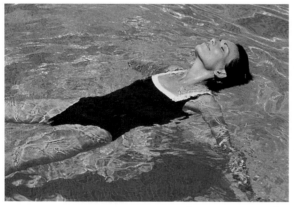

If you like to walk, play a sport, swim or ride a bike you'll be able to do it better by improving your breathing. If you find yourself getting tired easily or are stressed, you can improve matters with breathing techniques. You'll be surprised at how much your stamina and endurance both increase – and how quickly.

The basis of the training programme and the different exercises is to find out how you yourself feel – improving your mental and physical state is the aim of conscious breathing. Who is better equipped than you to find this out? Who is the better judge as to how far you can stretch yourself? Who knows better than you whether you can initiate changes and which should be chosen in any given situation? Only you. You are your best teacher.

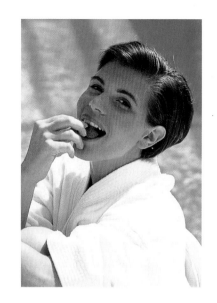

This book will systematically guide you on this path of learning and exercising. You will discover many ways to train your breathing in all its variations so you can increase the demands on yourself and make continuous progress. Breathing exercises provide you with the opportunity to enhance your everyday life, to meet its challenges with vitality.

With every exercise you will feel the power and freedom of breathing and of life itself. With one breath you will start each day afresh – you will breathe freely.

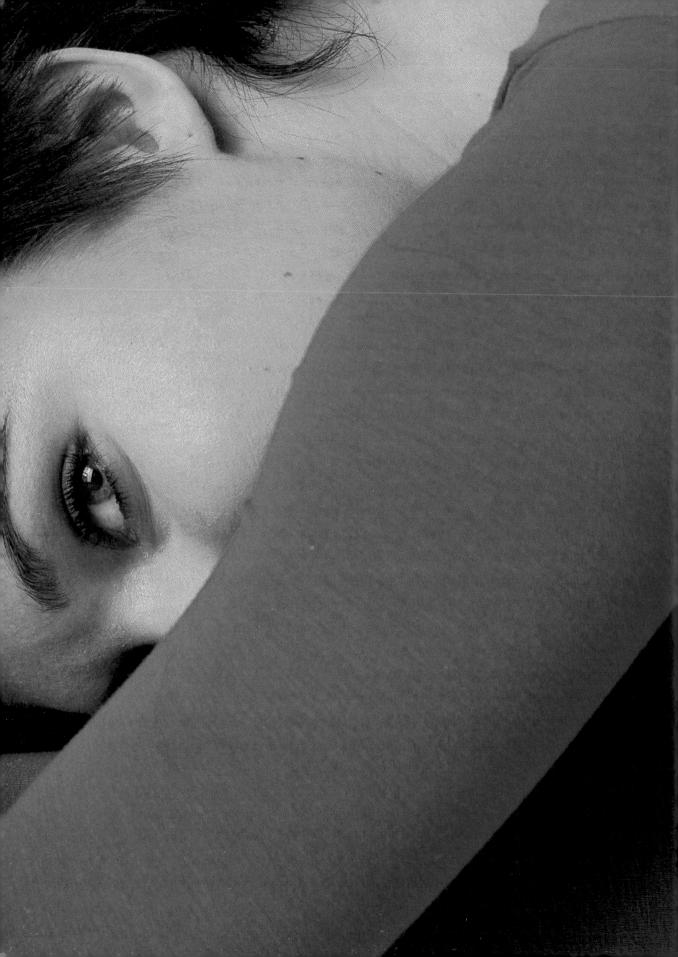

PART 1

A Guide to Breathing Freely

The key to good health is the efficient working of the cardiovascular system – the heart, lungs and blood circulation. Each relies on the other and they do their job so automatically that you hardly need think about it. Yet just one element is vital to all – air. To remain in prime condition at any age, you must power the system with your breathing, ensure that air flows unhindered to all parts of the body. To breathe freely you must make a conscious effort to control and shape your breath.

What you can achieve from this book

Breathing is the secret of constant rejuvenation. But to use it well, to discover its power, you need to become conscious of your breath. This original course of step-by-step exercises brings you closer to better health.

The most vital part of breath training is the experience of becoming aware of your own breathing. But it is helpful to have some understanding of the theory, to know more about the different parts of the body your breathing affects to make the training even more effective. All this is explained clearly through photographs and illustrations.

The exercises
There are 10 exercises, which lead you from discovering how your breath moves in your body (p. 38) through to feeling it as a wave washing through you (pp. 100–105). The exercises are designed to be done one after the other, as they appear in Part Two, and are formed into sequences. Each exercise starts from a basic position; these are conveniently grouped together (on pp. 20–31) so you can refer back to them any time.

The models have been photographed in leotards but these are not essential. What you need for effective exercising at home is explained on p. 18, and on p. 33 you will find suggestions for establishing a daily routine and sticking to it.

When you first start doing the exercises, allow 10 to 20 minutes for each session and concentrate on each one so you can fully appreciate the new breathing experience. Going slowly and calmly is the best way to absorb techniques which may be new to you and which you will need to practise before you feel their beneficial effects. You should also rest for a few minutes after a session before you get on with your daily life.

Your breathing
Exploring the sequences of each exercise will provide you with profound knowledge of your breathing. The time span for completing them is not important – the exercises can take as many weeks or months to master as you wish. You will always make progress.

When the breathing areas have been opened up and you mentally become aware of this, you will breathe on impulse which confirms that you have acquired a new kind of breathing. This is as important as the exercises themselves.

When you breathe on impulse your consciousness lets your body know that its general state has improved. This is positive information that will improve your memory. You will soon notice the sequences or sections you derive most benefit from and at which time of the day. Once you recognize an improvement in your breathing power, you can choose whether to do the exercises regularly or make up your own programme combining favourite sequences.

It is worth changing this from time to time so that you keep enjoying the exercises.

Your lifestyle
Having trained your breathing through these exercises you will feel the rewards in all you do every day. You will find you have greater stamina and increased well-being. In Part Three you will discover how to reap the benefits of breathing, from the moment you wake, to going to sleep. There are coping tactics for tension, little physical tricks to help you in challenging situations – either alone or in company. The secret power of it all is breathing.

If you have been ill or have physical problems, before you begin these exercises it may be best to discuss your intentions with your doctor. You will find a note on those exercises that may not be suitable for people with certain conditions.

Breathing awareness

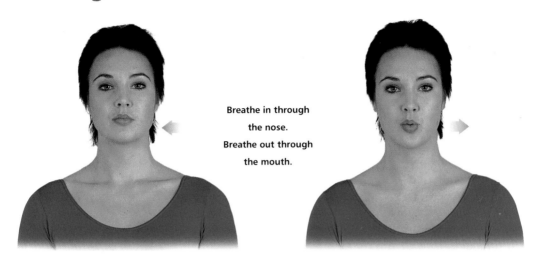

Breathe in through the nose. Breathe out through the mouth.

You start to breathe from birth and it becomes an automatic action. To discover the power of breathing, learning is involved, with mind and body working together. A baby learns by unconscious practising, doing something so many times it eventually becomes automatic. An adult can consciously learn one thing while doing another – an automatic action can become one you are aware of. This is particularly pertinent when you are learning something new.

Conscious learning

When you repeat an action you are aware of, you enhance your senses and become more alert. This is doubly stimulating – you shorten the process of practising because you act mechanically and consciously at the same time. Thinking about a movement before and while you are doing it forms the mental connection between mind and body. Breathing consciously establishes direct contact in the same way. After you have

exercised like this for a period of time it will take just a thought, one moment of concentration, to put you in direct touch with your breathing. The sooner you find how quickly this can be done the better it will be for your general well-being and for your inner self.

With the range of breathing techniques you will learn, it is possible to stimulate yourself mentally or calm yourself at will, helping you cope with everyday life. If you exercise while consciously thinking about what you are doing, it will encourage positive changes

in the way you breathe. If you concentrate on what you are doing, this will prevent you from exercising for too long because your brain will instantly register discomfort.

Assess your feelings

A combination of body and mind encourages you to assess how you feel – the state you are in – to achieve greater mobility, giving you endurance and strength. By repeating the exercises over and over again, this awareness will stay with you and your breathing. It is as if you are listening to yourself.

Breathing is catching

Make yourself aware of how other people breathe. If a person uses mainly abdominal breathing you will soon find it tiring to be in his or her company for any length of time. If you are with someone who breathes mainly through the chest, you will become nervous and agitated. You may even find yourself breathing just like them – you have been caught in their "breathing aura".

Your best protection is a balanced kind of breathing, with the air flowing into every breathing area of your body.

The way we breathe

Breathing is natural – we all do it. But do we do it to greatest advantage? To get air circulating around the body, it needs conscious effort and an understanding of the processes behind the power.

There are two ways in which air enters the body. The first is through the nose into the trachea (windpipe), the second is through the mouth into the trachea. It can leave either way.

Breathing in and out through the nose is the optimal process. It is calmer, slower and healthier when you are occupied with undemanding everyday activities. When air is taken in through the nose

● It is cleaned, warmed and moistened

● It takes its time to reach the trachea and thus the lungs. However, less air flows into the

body this way. With increased activity – when you need air quickly – you must breathe in through the mouth. When air is inhaled through the mouth:

● It travels a shorter distance

● There is less resistance

● The muscles have to work less hard in order to stimulate deep breathing.

You should always breathe through the mouth when you speak or sing because the breathing reflexes are faster and more impulsive. If you inhale through the nose there is simply not enough air coming in. If you pause too long – to "catch

your breath" – the flow of speech or rhythm of singing is interrupted.

When engaged in strenuous physical work (such as during childbirth, when a mother may pant or gasp) breathing through the mouth may be the best way to deal with the situation. You should make sure your jaws are not tensed, your teeth are at least a finger-width apart and your tongue is relaxed in the lower jaw. Your throat should be open so you inhale noiselessly.

When exhaling, the way through the nose is narrower and longer, so air emerges more slowly from the body and your breathing is calmer. Exhaling rapidly – in a "cleansing breath", for example, which prepares your lungs for the exercises to come, see p. 36 – is done through the mouth. You can slow down the breath even more when exhaling through the nose by humming (keep your lips closed).

Sniffing, as opposed to breathing through the nose, takes air in quickly; blowing sharply out through the nose can force stale air out of the lungs, preparing them for the arrival of new air.

The lungs are situated in breathing areas 3 and 4 (see pp. 16–17), protected by the ribcage. They are in a vacuum whose area changes according to the movement of the diaphragm, which causes the lungs to expand and contract.

The anatomy of the chest

When you breathe in, air enters the body through the nose ❶ or mouth ❷ and passes down the trachea (windpipe) ❸ into the lungs ❹. As the lungs expand, the ribs ❺ are pulled upward by the intercostal muscles ❻ between them, enlarging the chest area. The diaphragm ❼ contracts and the lungs fill with air. The heart ❽ pumps blood into the lungs, where it is re-oxygenated before being sent to the rest of the body.

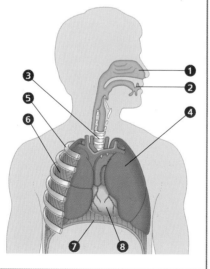

Breathing through the chest and abdomen

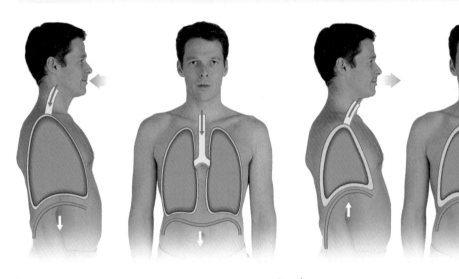

Breathing in – the diaphragm contracts   Breathing out – the diaphragm relaxes

The belief that you should "breathe with your abdomen" is widely supported. In fact, abdominal breathing is generally held to be preferable to thoracic respiration, or breathing through the chest.

But both these forms of breathing on their own are ineffectual – only some of the breathing muscles and only parts of the lungs are involved in the exchange of oxygen. The volume of the breath is reduced and you have to inhale more often. This is unnecessarily stressful for the body.

Combined effort

To breathe effectively you should combine abdominal and thoracic breathing so you use all the muscles and lung tissue you can. It is not enough to push out the stomach on the in-breath and pull it back on the out-breath. From the start of the training programme (see p. 38) you will experience how to feel your breath, a technique that will be deepened, expanded and strengthened in the sequences that follow. Once you achieve balanced breathing with the diaphragm, the effects can be felt in the abdomen, the back and the sides.

If the chest does not move during breathing, this leads to the other extreme – abdominal breathing only. There is insufficient or no activity in the chest and the diaphragm takes all the strain. If only (or mainly) the diaphragm is active the air only penetrates as far as the lower parts of the lungs and does not reach the large upper parts and the sides of the lungs.

People who breathe this way can be prone to depression and have little energy. If the intercostal muscles (see box, opposite) are not sufficiently activated, vitality is reduced and the body will show this as tiredness, leading to a state of exhaustion.

Shallow breathing

People under severe stress frequently breathe shallowly, inhaling and exhaling far too fast which increases the heart rate and subjects the body to even more stress.

Many asthma and chronic bronchitis sufferers use shallow breathing and also tend to have an elevated diaphragm so the lungs are not filled to capacity and the activity of the lung tissue is reduced even further. Air becomes scarce and the asthma or bronchitis attacks increase in frequency or severity.

The voice says a lot

It is common to find that people who use their voice a lot – but in the wrong way – also breathe shallowly. Their voices are often shrill and they tend to be continually short of breath. Such breathing leads to a susceptibility to colds and hoarseness, and can even cause harm to the vocal cords.

The effects of breath training

Wwhen you make the most of your breathing you will feel the effects from the inside out. Good breathing has a powerful and positive effect on the heart, circulation, immune system, organs, muscles and joints.

At the core of all the exercises in this book is the effect they have on your breathing. Through the very basic but invigorating act of taking in more air, your lungs will be cleansed and galvanized into increasing their capacity. By stimulating and strengthening your breathing muscles – the diaphragm and the intercostals between the ribs – your organs, heart and circulation will receive a new vitality.

The exercises are designed so that you will gradually experience an improvement in the functioning of all your organs as you train yourself with breathing. Your whole body will feel the benefits. The power of breathing carries vital oxygen via the blood to your muscles and this will in turn improve your mobility, as well as toning and strengthening the muscles themselves.

Within the sequences of each exercise are movements to improve your posture and mobility – which are essential to optimal breathing. At the beginning you will achieve this by following the sequences as they appear in the book, and

later, when more experienced, with a routine you can design for yourself as part of a regular daily activity.

As you do these exercises, your breathing, posture and mobility influence each other, and you will make progress on all fronts. You will also find a noticeable difference in your ability to concentrate because during the sequences you become very conscious of each movement – inside and around you. In fact, the power of your breathing combined with deep concentration will help you become more aware generally. With practice you will find it easier to "switch on" when your full attention is needed, and to "switch off" completely when you want to relax.

Know your breathing areas

These are the parts of your body with "elastic" walls, which means they can be affected by the movement of your breath. Breathe in and they expand, breathe out and they shrink back – the more exercise they get the better they work.

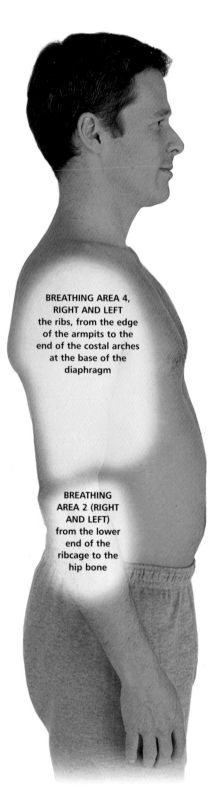

BREATHING AREA 4, RIGHT AND LEFT the ribs, from the edge of the armpits to the end of the costal arches at the base of the diaphragm

BREATHING AREA 2 (RIGHT AND LEFT) from the lower end of the ribcage to the hip bone

The breathing areas of the body

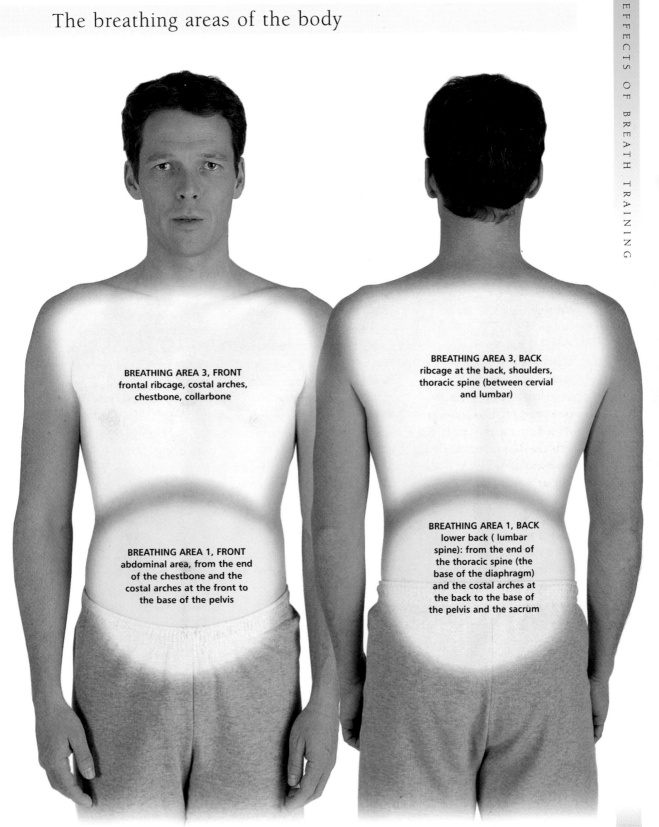

BREATHING AREA 3, FRONT
frontal ribcage, costal arches,
chestbone, collarbone

BREATHING AREA 3, BACK
ribcage at the back, shoulders,
thoracic spine (between cervial
and lumbar)

BREATHING AREA 1, FRONT
abdominal area, from the end
of the chestbone and the
costal arches at the front to
the base of the pelvis

BREATHING AREA 1, BACK
lower back (lumbar
spine): from the end of
the thoracic spine (the
base of the diaphragm)
and the costal arches at
the back to the base of
the pelvis and the sacrum

Effective exercising

Getting into the habit of exercising is the way to increased vitality, to balance and harmony. For maximum effect, you should establish a daily exercise routine on which you can build an on-going programme.

When you have discovered the power of breathing through effective exercising you will feel a general – and noticeable – improvement in your well-being. It could be because hyperactivity, connected with shallow breathing, is reduced, or because previously inefficient breathing becomes more active, making you more alert.

By knowing how to breathe properly, you achieve balance and harmony, leading to a continuous increase in physical and mental power – and new vitality. In this book you will discover two basic exercise types. The first, experience exercises, use breathing for everyday vitalizing and calming. They are simple to do, offer immediate help to make you more awake and stimulated, to banish tension or cope with fatigue. You will find these in Part Three (pp. 106–125).

The second type, in Part Two (pp. 38–105), are strengthening exercises. They have a different dimension. They are structured for continuity, the first two showing new ways of breathing and the other eight helping you build up the power. These exercises present a challenge, open up new possibilities and guarantee step-by-step progress.

In the next few pages you will find the basic positions which introduce you to breath training when you are standing, sitting or lying down. You will find these techniques most useful in everyday situations – such as travelling long distances, or having to stand for a long time. They are also the starting points for the 10 sets of strengthening exercises which help you to get to know yourself and your body.

Self assessment
Run through some questions in your mind:
- Do I feel alert or tired?
- Can I feel my breath?
- How am I breathing?
- Can I feel the breath in parts of my body?
- Is my posture good or bad?
- Are my muscles tense?

When you have registered how your mind and body feel – and made contact with what needs to be put right – you should warm up a little to prepare your muscles for the activity to come. After this you can start on your own personal training programme.

What you will need
The exercises in this book are personal to you. You do them in the quiet and calm of your own home, in your own time.

Clothing: The models are shown in exercise clothes but you can wear what you like so long as it is comfortably loose. Trousers with a tight-fitting waistband are inappropriate but any casual clothing – even pyjamas – will do so long as it is will keep you warm. It is important not to feel cold, especially when you are doing the slow exercises. If you begin to sweat because you have increased the pace of the exercises it will not do you any harm so long as there are no draughts in the room.

The place: Choose a room that is warm and has space for you to move freely. Collect together all you need before you begin so the continuous flow of the exercises will not be interrupted because you have to fetch something you have forgotten.

Equipment: For the exercises you do lying down you should have a floor covering which protects you from getting cold and provides moderate support for your back. A gym mat is ideal, but you could also use a thick blanket or a thick-pile rug. Bare floorboards are unsuitable as you must feel comfortable when lying down. Some soft cushions or a rolled towel might come in handy for extra comfort under vulnerable areas – the head, neck, shoulders or legs.

For those exercises you do sitting, choose a chair or stool with a moderately hard seat. A soft or springy seat is not suitable; you must have a little resistance. The height of the seat should be the length of your lower leg (from the sole of to the knee) when your feet rest flat on the floor. It can be a little lower but should not be higher.

Fresh air: Fresh, oxygen-rich air is your body's most important food. It is food you can do without for only a short time. Let it into the room before you start – open the windows, make sure there is enough humidity (use a humidifier when the heating is on). You want to avoid draughts so if the window is open make sure the door of the room is closed.

Peace and quiet: Shut out all unnecessary noise while doing your breathing exercises as it will affect your concentration. Put the answerphone on, or turn the ringing volume right down, so that your session won't be interrupted.

Time: Allow between 10 and 20 minutes a day at the start, increasing it as you get used to the exercises.

Finishing a session

When you have finished each day's exercises try to note any changes, even if they seem insignificant, in a daily diary. Slowly raise yourself into a sitting position, stay seated for a moment and take a few slow breaths. You are looking for changes in your breathing, posture and the tone of your muscles. Very slowly get on to your feet and once again see if you feel anything different.

CHECKLIST

Before you start
• Air the room well
• Wear loose, comfortable clothes
• Collect together everything you need
• Chose the right time of the day
• Do not exercise on a full stomach
• Cut out distracting noises.

The right way to exercise
• Warm up (p. 37)
• Make sure you know how you feel in yourself
• Concentrate
• Be determined to continue
• Set a reasonable time and moderate challenges
• Make a note of the changes you feel have occurred.

After the exercises
You should feel stimulated and well – if you are tired you probably exercised at the wrong time of day or for too long. Change your routine.

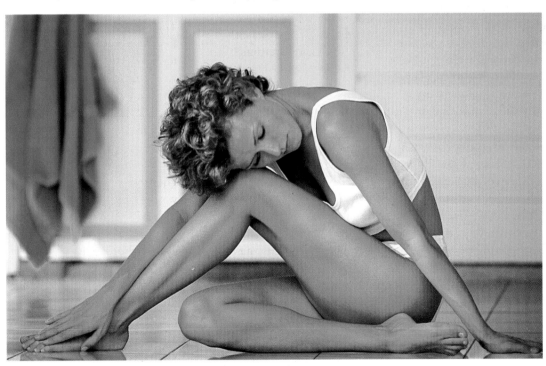

The basics for all exercises

You will meet the positions described in this chapter time and time again as you practise, so it is a good idea to become familiar with them before you start. They form the basis for the exercises and their sequences in Part Two of the book and they are grouped together as a useful reference guide you can consult at any time.

Standing positions

Basic

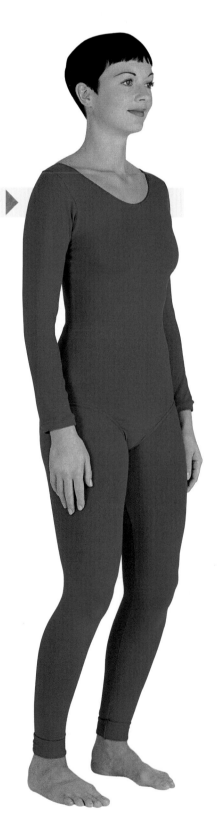

1 Stand with the soles of your feet – the heels, balls and big toes – flat on the floor. The weight of your body should be equally distributed on the soles.

2 Keep your knees slightly bent. Straight knees can have an adverse effect on the spine and pelvis as can bending them too much. If either is advised in an exercise it is because your body will be warmed up and ready.

3 Keep your pelvis centered, neither bent backward nor forward. Check whether it is in the correct position by placing your hands, palms downward, on the base of your spine and the pubic bone. Move your pelvis about until it rests in a position that is comfortable. This position might change during the exercises.

4 Your spine naturally curves in an S shape. Stretch it slightly from the base of the spine to the top of your head. Your neck will automatically be stretched when you do this. Keep your shoulders broad and relaxed, with your arms hanging loose.

The rule is: When you breathe while standing up you must feel the movement of the breath in your pelvis. Your weight rests on the physical centre of gravity, a little below the navel.

The Basic position affects your posture.

With the help of breathing you will gradually acquire the correct upright position, by adjusting the position of your bones and by balancing and strengthening your muscles. Your pelvis is affected by your posture and you should ensure that the position it is in feels natural even when it changes. Do not change it by tightening the muscles of the stomach, hips and buttocks – this leads to reduced breathing activity in the abdominal area. Adjust it by balancing your weight on your soles.

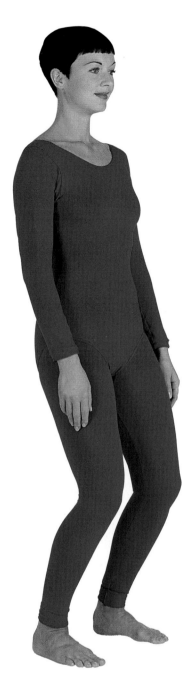

Wide-hipped

1 Stand with your feet hip-width apart, or even slightly wider, with knees slightly bent. You should be relaxed and feel no strain on your back, shoulders or neck.

2 Keep your feet parallel, with the toes neither flopping inward nor outward. Let your arms hang loosely by your side.

The rule is: The weight of your body should be equally carried by both feet. In order to make sure this is the case, shift the weight from one foot to the other without lifting the soles of your feet until you can feel they are equal.

The Wide-hipped position affects balance.

If you are comfortable and relaxed you can stand like this for some time. Your weight is taken by both your feet and you feel quite secure.

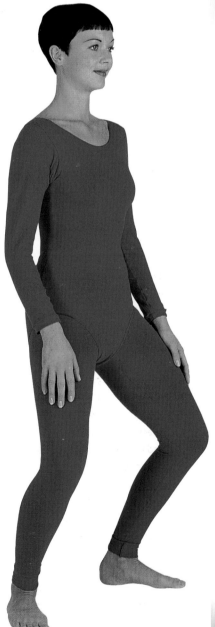

Straddled legs

1 Similar to the Wide-hipped position (above), but in this one the feet are much further apart, pointing outward, and the knees are bent a little more.

2 Stand with your feet as wide apart as is comfortable – without feeling strain. Rest your hands on your thighs.

The Straddled legs position affects balance.

The equal distribution of your body's weight on the soles of your feet gives you stability.

The rule is: Find what's right for you. Your ability may differ from somebody else's, and can depend on how fit you are. Be sure not to stand on something slippery when in this position.

21

Rider's

1 Similar to the Straddled legs position (p. 21), but in this one the knees are bent more. Your soles should be flat on the floor. Do not bend your knees to such an extent that the heels rise; the weight of your body should still rest on both feet.

2 Keep your trunk straight, not rounded or hollowed, elbows resting on knees. It is easy to feel the movement of your breath when you are in this position.

The rule is: Imagine you are a jockey riding your horse to the winning post. Your buttocks are lifted from the saddle, your upper body is aligned with the horse's neck. This becomes easier with daily practice.

The Rider's position affects the leg, buttocks and hip muscles.

At first you may find it a strain to remain like this for long, but you will be aware of the increase in the power of your muscles every time you practise.

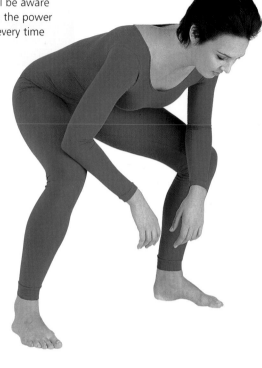

Standing coachman

1 Take up the Rider's position but bend your knees slightly more, bend your trunk forward and rest your forearms on your thighs. Your elbows should point outward, your chest should be open, your shoulders wide.

2 Stay in this position for a while, calmly breathing in and out in the direction of the floor and inhaling slowly through your nose.

The rule is: Make sure that the weight of your body is resting on the soles of your feet. You should clearly feel your breath in breathing area 1 (see explanation on p. 17).

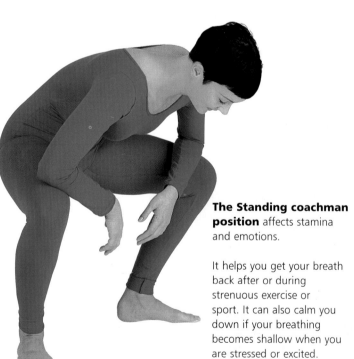

The Standing coachman position affects stamina and emotions.

It helps you get your breath back after or during strenuous exercise or sport. It can also calm you down if your breathing becomes shallow when you are stressed or excited.

Squatting position

Birthing

1 Squat very low, with your feet more than hip-width apart. You may find it easy to place your soles flat on the floor, but if you can't it doesn't matter. It is sufficient to rest on the balls of your feet with slightly lifted heels.

2 If you find it difficult to balance at first, place both hands on the seat of a chair. Move slightly backward when inhaling while shifting your heels to the floor. Do this until you can take your hands off the chair. Breathe in and out a few times and get up as soon as it feels uncomfortable.

The rule is: Feel so relaxed you could carry on a conversation.

The Birthing position affects your feelings, being both calming and stabilizing.

You don't have to get into this position often but while you are in it your breath moves rapidly down and activates the organs in the lower abdominal areas.

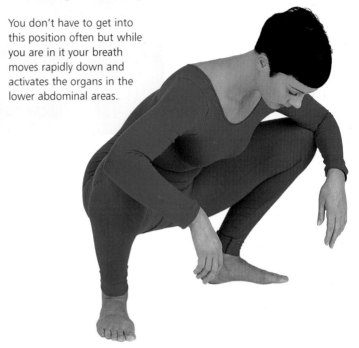

Kneeling positions

Sphinx

1 Kneel on your mat or cushion, place your insteps flat on the floor and sit on your heels. Your trunk should be straight.

2 Place one hand on each thigh. If your insteps or knees feel taut place a cushion between your heels and buttocks. Breathe evenly.

The rule is: Your whole body should feel very relaxed in this position. Keep the cushions that help you feel comfortable within reach as this is an excellent position to rest in for a while between exercises.

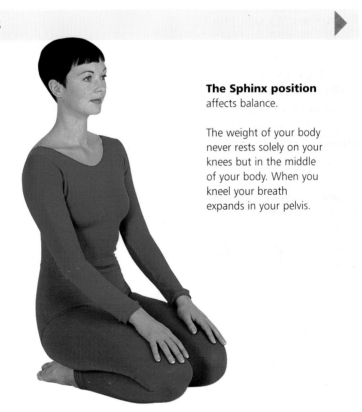

The Sphinx position affects balance.

The weight of your body never rests solely on your knees but in the middle of your body. When you kneel your breath expands in your pelvis.

Crouching

1 Sit on your heels, bend your trunk forward and rest it on your thighs. Let your forehead touch the floor if you like.

2 You can rest your arms at your sides, or in front of you, or cross them, clasping opposite elbows, and place them under your forehead. Try all these until you find the most comfortable.

The rule is: Feel very relaxed. Crouching is a good resting position between exercises.

The Crouching position affects your breathing areas.

If your arms rest by your sides the breath in breathing area 1 is stimulated, if they are in front of you breathing areas 1 and 4 are stimulated (see pp. 16–17).

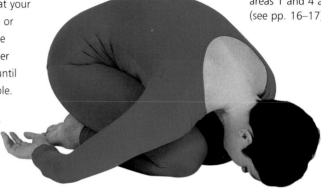

On all fours

1 With your knees hip-width apart, kneel on your mat or cushion. Bend your trunk forward with your hands on the floor, level with your shoulders, with your fingertips pointing forward. Your back should be straight, not hollowed or rounded.

2 Keep your head aligned with your spine and check that your body weight is equally distributed on knees and hands.

3 Breathe out and pull in your stomach, then let go of your stomach as you breathe in. Do this four times in quick succession.

4 Keeping your back and head straight, breathe out and rest your weight on your right hand and left knee. As you breathe in, shift your weight so it is carried equally by both hands and knees. Breathe out and lift right hand and left knee slightly off the floor.

5 Breathe in and shift your weight back to both hands and knees. Breathe out and move your weight to the left hand and right knee. Shift your weight a few times in this way changing from one opposing side to the other. Rest on all fours in between.

The rule is: Shifting your weight diagonally across your body increases your stability.

The On All Fours position affects your energy levels and balance.

This exercise will boost you when you are feeling tired and is a good position for stabilizing and exercising your back muscles, and increasing your sense of balance (see pp. 16–17).

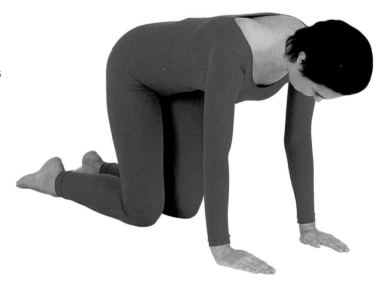

Sitting positions

King's

1 Sit on a chair with your legs in front of you, hip-width apart, and your soles flat on the floor. Place your hands in the middle of your thighs.

2 Shift your weight from one buttock to the other, moving gently until you can feel some resistance from your "sitting bones". Balance your weight on those bones until you feel comfortable. Move around on your buttocks, forward and backward, and rotate your pelvis.

3 As soon as you can feel the flow of energy from the soles of your feet to your calves and upward to your thighs, stretch your trunk a little each time you breathe in and support yourself on your heels at the same time. The energy will gradually expand into your pelvis. Breathe out and let go of the tension. Breathe in again, and feel the flow surging along your spine.

4 With each breath, the flow of energy will move up your body – from the pelvis to half way up the spine, then to the top of the spine. Every time you inhale, stretch the trunk a little further. Repeat this exercise up to five times until you are perfectly upright. Relax your shoulders.

The rule is: Find the right position for your weight to rest on your pelvis. This ensures that the rest of the trunk, the chest, shoulders and neck will automatically adjust themselves.

Note: Having found the correct position, you should not force yourself to keep it. Your pelvis should still have some mobility. It will help if you support yourself on your legs and feet so they carry your weight. Actively involving your legs and feet is an important part of the King's position.

The King's position affects posture and well-being.

Sitting like this gives a relaxed, unslumped posture and allows your breath to expand freely in each of the breathing areas. Every breath will stimulate you – from the base of your spine to the parting of your hair. You will feel alert and well balanced, able to think and act calmly.

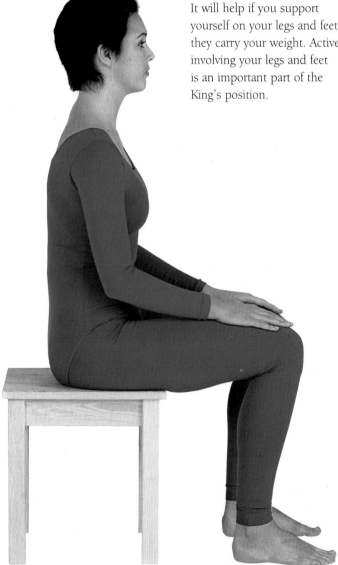

Seated coachman

1 Sit in the King's position but with your legs further apart.

2 Bend your trunk forward and place your elbows on your thighs, slightly above the knees. Do not put any of your body weight on to your elbows. Your weight should rest in the middle of your body supported by your legs. Your spine and neck should remain stretched while you are in this position and when breathing in and out.

The rule is: Feel your breath expand to the base of your spine when you inhale. You can enforce this by pushing the base of your spine down on to the seat of the chair and inhaling in the direction of your lumbar spine.

The Seated coachman position affects your spine and abdominal wall.

This position is good for resting between exercises. It also relaxes your abdominal wall and regenerates your lumbar spine. If you spend a lot of time sitting down, do this exercise to ensure vital oxygen reaches your spine.

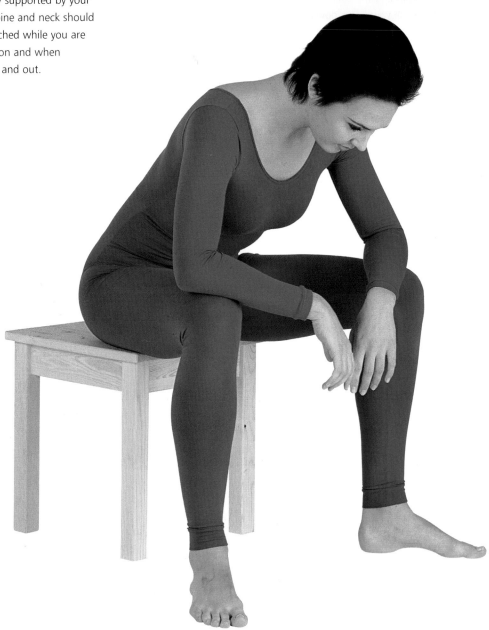

Cross-legged

1 Sit on the floor with your legs crossed and your body weight resting firmly on the floor. Your knees do not have to touch the floor – only very flexible people can do this.

2 Place your hands on your knees for some resistance and breathe in deeply. Pause, then exhale and push your knees down slightly. Continue in this way until your knees are as far apart as possible without causing the groin to tense up – this restricts the flow of your breath.

Note: If you find this position uncomfortable, try placing the soles of your feet against each other with your knees apart.

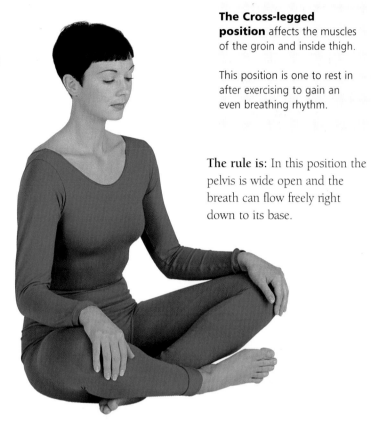

The Cross-legged position affects the muscles of the groin and inside thigh.

This position is one to rest in after exercising to gain an even breathing rhythm.

The rule is: In this position the pelvis is wide open and the breath can flow freely right down to its base.

Thinking

1 Sit on the floor with your legs wide apart. With your back slightly rounded, the weight of your body is carried by your pelvis.

2 Rest your arms on your knees and breathe freely and evenly.

The rule is: Become calm and relaxed so you think more clearly and your concentration is improved.

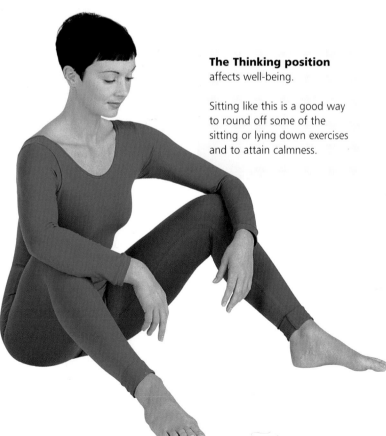

The Thinking position affects well-being.

Sitting like this is a good way to round off some of the sitting or lying down exercises and to attain calmness.

Lying positions

Supine

1 Lie on your back with your knees and feet loose and hands by your sides. This is the starting position for several exercises and good for resting.

2 If you feel there is too much tension in your neck put a small cushion under your head or a rolled towel under your neck so you feel comfortable. Breathe evenly in and out.

The rule is: Feel very relaxed without any apparent tension in any part of your body.

Note: Stretching your legs too far while in the Supine position is not advised. It can cause leg and foot muscles to cramp, as well as a build up of tension in the lumbar spine – a problem area for people who have sedentary occupations.

The Supine position affects your feelings of well-being.

Being able to relax without any tension is the first step to falling asleep.

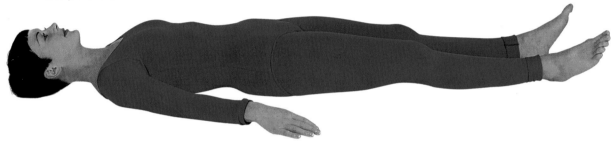

Dune

1 Lie on your back with your knees bent and hip-width apart, the soles of your feet resting flat on the floor. Your pelvis will rise a little in this position, taking the weight off your lumbar spine which automatically moves closer to the floor. This allows the diaphragm to fill the breathing areas at the back, creating space in breathing area 1 (see p. 17) which you should be able to feel.

2 Place your arms at your sides, slightly away from your body. Lower your spine every time you breathe out – imagine you are sinking into the ground as if you were lying on soft sand. This stimulates breathing in the back. You can help this slight movement of your pelvis and spine by gently pressing your heels into the floor. Make sure there is no additional tension building up in the abdomen when you exhale.

3 Place your hands lightly on top of your abdomen to check that as you breathe it rises and falls without being forced.

The rule is: Use as a warm up for the exercises and as a way of relaxing between them.

The Dune position affects the lower parts of your back.

This is a restful position for the lumbar spine.

Package

1 Lie on your back and use your hands to pull your knees up to your chest. Your elbows should be just far enough from your body to keep your shoulders relaxed.

2 Make sure your head and neck are comfortable, using a pillow or neck roll for support if necessary. You should not feel tension in these areas.

3 Breathe out and pull your legs closer to your chest. Breathe in and move your legs back to their original position, without taking your hands off your knees. Repeat a few times and give in to the slight stretching you will feel in your back. Then inhale and exhale again in a position in which the distance of your legs to your chest feels comfortable. This is a resting position.

The Package position affects all muscles in the back, especially the lower back, giving the discs more space and taking the strain off the spine.

You will find this a good way to relax after fitness training or after having exercised your back muscles.

The rule is: The elbows must point away from the body otherwise the breathing in the walls of the diaphragm – breathing area 4 – will be restricted. If the elbows are close to the body you will be inclined to hunch your shoulders.

An alternative position

You may find it easier to do this exercise without holding on to your knees. In this case make sure your arms are not too close to your body so they keep you balanced. When you move your knees toward your chest you can find the position that is most comfortable for your arms.

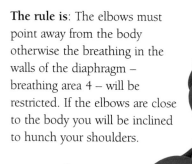

Foot pressure

In the exercises you will sometimes be asked to put pressure on your foot (or feet) as a means of supporting yourself. You must apply just enough weight to the sole of one or both feet for you to feel the pressure move gently from your feet to your legs, up to your pelvis and to the trunk.

You will need to try it a few times (as described in the King's position on p. 25) to find out exactly how much pressure is necessary. Too much pressure

will make your legs and the lower part of the abdomen tense. If the pressure is correct – on the soles and not the balls of your feet – you will have the feeling that you are being "carried".

The pressure should vary according to the tension in your muscles. In the course of your daily exercising you will notice these changes clearly and quickly learn how to move your heels, balls and toes to adjust the pressure.

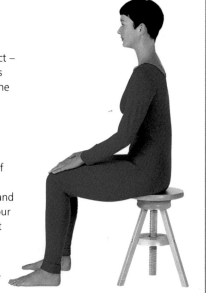

Rolling the vertebrae

This technique involves opening up the spine – from one vertebra to the next – so that it becomes mobile and flexible. It is an exercise to do slowly and gently so the muscles in the back are stretched. You should be careful not to tense up. The steps show how to start at the top with the cervical vertebrae, moving on to the thoracic and finishing with the lumbar. Then, from a fully bent position, you roll upward from the sacrum. Read about the spine's anatomy (right) and as you breathe out slowly imagine the number of vertebrae in the area being rolled.

1 Stand in the basic position, with legs slightly bent and feet hip-width apart. Breathe out three times and begin to roll.

2 Bend over and breathe in, then in one slow out-breath roll all the vertebrae in one part of the spine. Let your arms hang loosely.

3 Do the exercise slowly, adjusting your rolling movement to the rhythm of your breath. After rolling several vertebrae, breathe in.

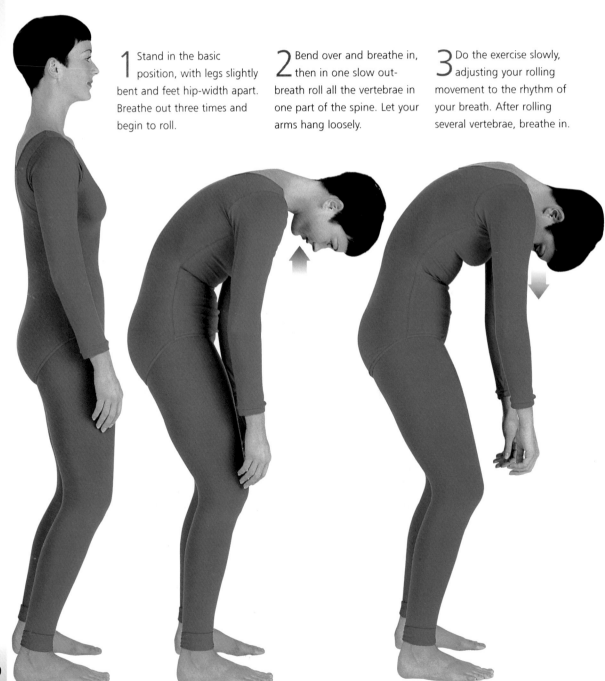

Rolling your vertebrae is an excellent warm up exercise. You can concentrate on the vertebrae that are tense. This improves the circulation to your spine and can prevent your back from getting tired.

4 When you feel ready to move on, breathe out and bend your body further. Continue until each section of the spine has been rolled.

The anatomy of the spine

The spinal column is a combination of bones and fluid which support the body and permit a wide range of movement. Vertebrae are found along the whole length of the spine which is divided into four.

Cervical spine. Seven vertebrae – the smallest – in the neck.

Thoracic spine. 12 vertebrae which form the upper back and connect to the 12 pairs of ribs.

Lumbar spine. Five vertebrae – the largest – which carry most of the body's weight.

In these three parts each vertebra is separated from its neighbour by an intervertebral disc which absorbs shock and cushions against jarring.

Sacrum and coccyx. The tail end, where vertebrae are fused together.

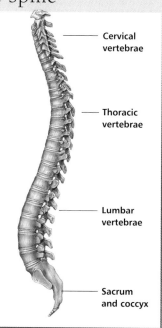

- Cervical vertebrae
- Thoracic vertebrae
- Lumbar vertebrae
- Sacrum and coccyx

5 Now roll yourself upright in the same way. As a daily exercise, do it both ways slowly and then do it fast. Repeat two to three times.

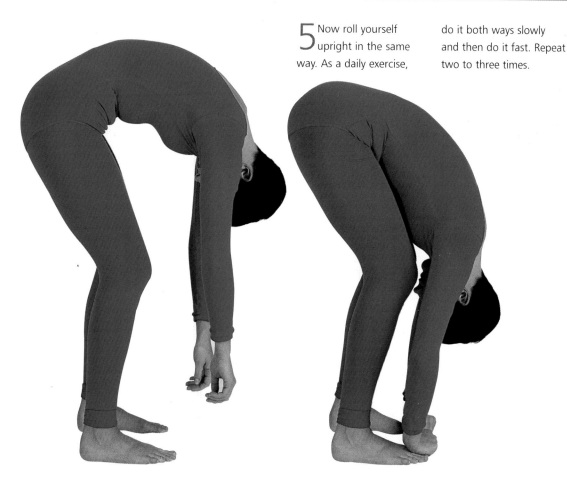

31

About the exercises

The aim of each exercise is to improve your breathing and to enable you to track it so well that you do it without wasting any energy. Through repetition you act in a way that soon will seem wholly natural.

All the physical movements you do every day have become automatic through learning and practice. When you walk you don't have to think about putting one foot in front of the other. If you had to concentrate on this and the other natural things you do, as well as going about your daily life, you would be exhausted.

Automatic – well-practised – actions make life easier. The new sensations you experience when you start to improve your breathing technique through this range of exercises will open up new dimensions to actions you had previously taken for granted.

Most of our most elementary actions are learned in the first year or so of life. Consider, for example, reaching and holding. At first a baby just misses the object he wants to hold. He keeps on trying and finally the complex interplay of muscles and nerves involved work together. Whenever he attempts this action the brain registers what happens and the what he did becomes an experience which remains with him.

The same thing happens when a baby learns how to grip. He first becomes aware of the object, then by involving many groups of muscles extends the arm until he reaches the object he wants. Just like the baby, each time you exercise particular muscles for a reason you find it easier to do.

The more opportunities a baby has to repeat an action the quicker he will manage to do it perfectly, and the more confident he will become. The muscles now act automatically, leaving him free to concentrate on the next steps of learning, to move on.

This is a simple example of one stage in human development and it is just the beginning. Experience can always be widened. Studies conducted over many years have shown that learning and practising elementary actions highly stimulates the brain. Children who are encouraged to learn and practise what they have learned are more alert and have a quicker understanding of things than children who are not mentally stimulated.

We can follow the example of artists – in the broadest sense, people who know their profession, never stop trying to improve, are always interested and ready to learn something new. It's the secret of vitality.

Programming your muscles

Movement is carried out as a conscious action – that is, accompanied by certain thoughts. When you imagine a certain movement, the tone of the muscle is pre-programmed by the brain and nervous system. A movement prepared in this way is easier to do.
Try this experiment. Sit at a table with your forearms on the table, palms down. When you feel that both arms are resting comfortably imagine that you are lifting your right forearm but don't move it. Imagine lifting it three or four times. Then briefly lift it and put it on the table again.

Immediately lift your left arm without imagining it first and put it back on the table.

Even with a movement as small as this you will notice the difference in the weight you are lifting. Your right arm will seem lighter than the left one.

With any exercise, thinking about it before you start will pay dividends. When you carry out the movement you will notice the difference.

Establishing a routine

Like most things that are good for you, breath training takes time and effort. Rewards come soonest when you've set up a routine and stick to it

How long you exercise is up to you. A lot will depend on your ability to concentrate. You should also enjoy exercising and find it interesting or it won't have the desired effect. A session should last for at least 5 minutes and not longer than 30 minutes without a break, including time for warming up. The given time on an exercise is the average time it will take once you have become familiar with it.

Depending on what you have chosen for the day's routine – whether a whole exercise, or a few sequences of it – it is always important that you pay close attention to your breath and its movements.

Your breath is as individual as yourself. You will experience something new every day during the course of your training. Your breath will grow and gain in calmness, vitality and strength.

Try to exercise at the same time each day so that it becomes a habit. If you exercise in the morning, you will soon notice that the day will go better. If you exercise in the evening, you will find an increase in energy. Try to choose a time of day that meets all the criteria – time, air, lack of noise, certainly no interruptions (see pp. 18–19).

Some people are ready to exercise and are more perceptive in the morning. But if your mornings are hectic, choose the late afternoon, or when you come home from work. You will soon notice that you are re-energized and enjoy the rest of the day instead of feeling fatigued and only able to do what is absolutely essential. Some people might find it easier to do two short sessions, in the morning and the afternoon.

Avoid exercising after a meal. A full stomach has a negative effect on your breathing. Your circulation is concentrating on digesting the food you've eaten, leaving little energy for anything else.

Set yourself challenges

Exercising means making continuous progress so that every day you move on a little. Every time you challenge your body, your breathing and your concentration you gain inner and outer strength. You need a little discipline, too. There will be days when you find it difficult. But don't give in. Do your daily exercises even if you have to "force" yourself. You will be surprised at how full of vitality you will be even though you felt tired at the start. At such times choose the exercises you know well and have done often. On those days when you are feeling strong and energetic, try an exercise you have been meaning to tackle, or work out a new programme. In other words adjust to how you feel. Don't demand too much of yourself on good days by exercising too much. You should never get out of breath as this weakens your memory and your body's defences. If it happens, stop the exercise and breathe evenly in and out until you are rested, then continue.

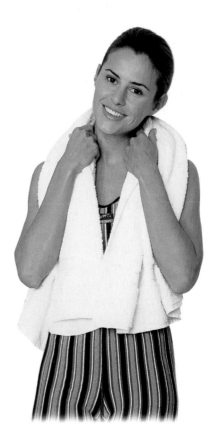

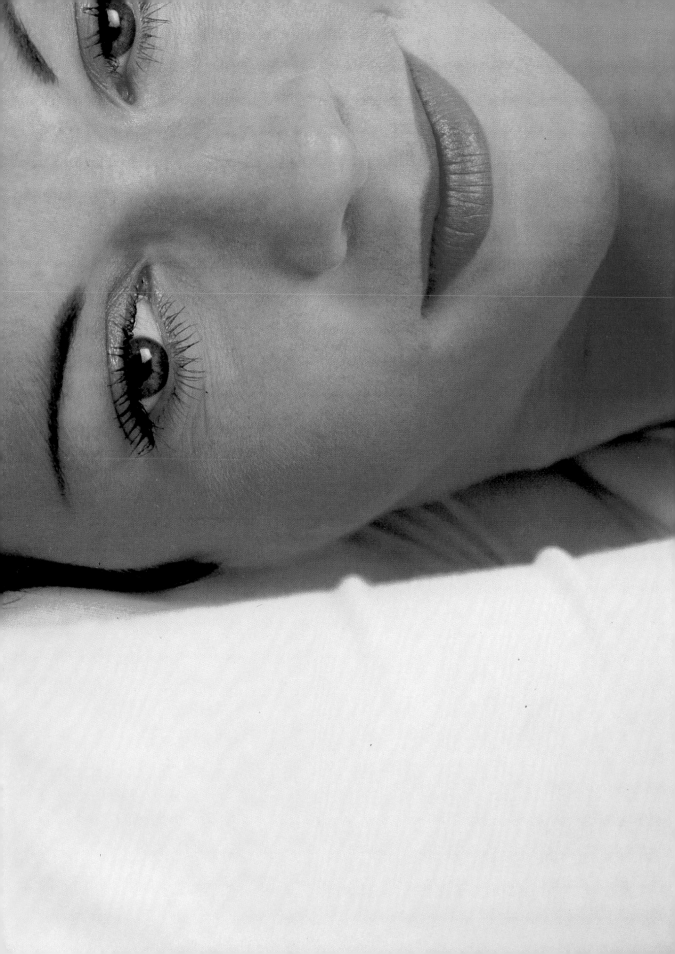

PART 2
The Exercises

This section comprises an enjoyable series of exercises designed to build your strength and stamina and improve your general well-being. The first two will teach you how to breathe and how to feel your breath as a power surge in your body. After this are eight exercises, each containing several sequences to condition your muscles, from which you will learn to appreciate the effects of being aware of every breath you take.

Discover the power of breathing

To make the most of breathing it is necessary to know how it's done, and how breath moves within the body. If you are relaxed you can follow its continuous movement, which both shapes you and is shaped by you.

You will find exactly how breath moves in the body as you progress through the various exercises. But before you start on them, you need to warm up and prepare yourself with a few basic activities.

Because the way the air flows inside you can change – it can become more or less intense, with a greater or lesser volume – you have to learn to listen to your breath and try to understand it. This requires you to become aware of yourself and your surroundings and to be able to concentrate on the movement of air within you. A calm and quiet place, where no one can intrude, is best for this.

Clear the nose

To breathe well your nose needs to be clear so air can flow unhindered. It is not just the common cold that blocks the nasal passage – polluted air can deposit tiny particles on the sensitive lining, or an allergy may cause excess mucus. So first blow your nose (gently), then beat your fingertips lightly along the bridge of your nose and the sinuses (follow the bone under your eyes). If you hum at the same time it will dislodge anything adhering to the lining.

The cleansing breath

The first step of every breathing exercise, the cleansing breath prepares the lungs for the exchange of oxygen about to take place, so that clean air can be transported to all the organs of the body via the blood and the millions of cells can receive essential nutrients. To make room for clean air in the lungs, a large amount of stale air has to be exhaled. Because most people haven't been taught how to breathe well, a little stale air always remains in the lungs, causing them to become slack and not as elastic as they should be. The cleansing breath – deep out-breathing – removes it. Either of the following methods

will clear the lungs of stale air. Breathe in through the nose and out through the mouth, but do not do it too much or too vigorously as it can lead to hyperventilation.

Method 1: Breathe out as vigorously as you can, letting your body bend forward just a little. Pull in your abdominal muscles while, at the same time, applying a little pressure to your ribs with your hands so that it forces the air out of the lungs. Pull yourself upright as you breathe in – but only take in as much air as feels natural. Do this two or three times – any more could put a strain on

your circulation and you will feel dizzy. If this happens, you have allowed in excessive quantities of air.

Method 2: You can also cleanse your breath by breathing out vigorously and swinging your arms forward as you do so. Breathe in and swing your arms back over your head in a semicircle. Repeat three to five times but do not exaggerate the movements too much.

Note: As your breathing becomes more efficient you will only need to breathe deeply in either of these ways once before you start exercising.

Warming up

The purpose of warming up is to stimulate the circulation so your body is ready for the exercises to come. The simple movements here are also quite refreshing in their own right and will give you a boost at any time. Stand by an open window if you can and benefit from the fresh air.

Stretch away

Start the warm-up by stretching your arms and legs and yawning. Do this for several minutes until you start to feel warm.

Tap arms and legs

Keep your hands relaxed and use a light consistent touch. Start tapping along one hand, up the arm to the shoulder then as far down the back as you can reach. Do the other arm in the same way. Do the legs next, working both hands together. As you breathe out, start at the outside of the hips and tap down to the feet. Then, breathing in, tap up the legs to the thighs.

Tap your trunk

Make relaxed fists. Starting at the chestbone tap toward the shoulders along each collarbone. Bend slightly forward then use your fists to tap your back in breathing area 1 (the lumbar region), moving your hands as high up as possible – to the diaphragm if you can.

Shake it up

Shake one arm at a time from the shoulder, which must be relaxed. Let go all the tension when you breathe out. You will feel a slight tingling in your arm. Do the same with your legs, one at a time, shaking from the hip.

Make circles

A great refresher when sitting at a desk, in a car, on a plane or train journey. Simply make circles with your hands and feet, from the wrists and ankles, first one way then the other.

Follow the arrows

In the exercises that follow you will find arrows which indicate the recommended breathing at various stages.

◀ Blue arrow **inhale**
▶ Red arrow **exhale**

▲ Blue arrow and red arrow
▼ **breathe freely in and out**

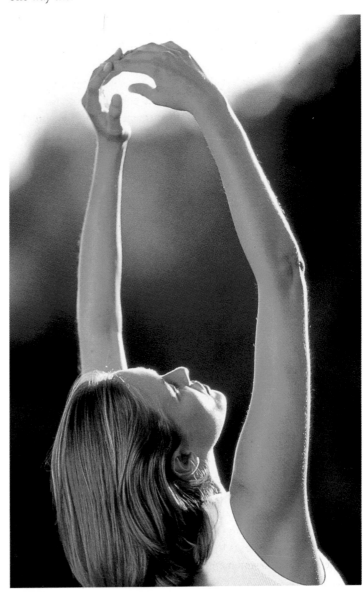

Starting
position –
King's
page 25

Become aware of your breathing. . .1

1 Place your palms on your trunk, at the top of the ribcage with fingertips meeting in the middle of the chest. The idea is to move your palms slowly away from the centre to follow the walls of the diaphragm to the sides. Move your palms at your own pace as you breathe in, pause and breathe out.

Note: An exercise to introduce you to your breathing and the way breath moves in your body. It has two sequences, each of which should take about 5 minutes, and is best done in the evening. You should feel calm, be aware, feel happy to be going on an adventure of discovery. The end result will be deep effective natural breathing, and you will have learned more about your body.

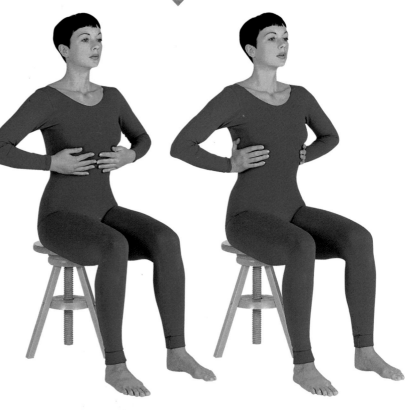

2 When you have reached the walls of the ribcage at your sides, move your palms downward in the same way to the middle of your body so you can feel how your abdomen moves. You will notice that it rises and expands with each in-breath and falls and shrinks with each out-breath.

3 Move your palms along your body between your ribcage and pelvis – this is called the abdominal area. Now place your hands just above the waist at your sides and breathe deeply in and out two or three times. Try to follow the movement of your breath inside you when you are doing this. See if, in your thoughts, you can accompany the breath you've just taken and visualize it flowing to the area you have just explored with your hands. This is called breathing on impulse.

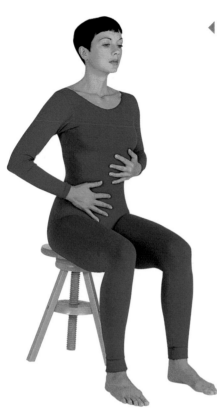

◀ 4 Place your left hand at the base of the diaphragm, the right one on the lower ribs so you feel the lower costal arches under your palm. Try to follow the movement of your breath inside the chest area. You will feel the costal arches move a little to the side and upward each time you breathe in and sink back when you breathe out. Change hand positions and repeat, adjusting the palm pressure until you feel your breath clearly.

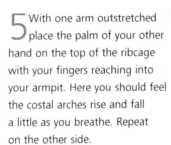

5 With one arm outstretched ▶ place the palm of your other hand on the top of the ribcage with your fingers reaching into your armpit. Here you should feel the costal arches rise and fall a little as you breathe. Repeat on the other side.

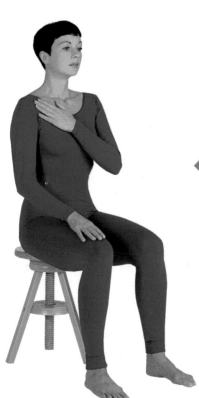

◀ 6 With one hand on your thigh, place the palm of your other hand alongside your collarbone. Move your palm down your chest to the base of your diaphragm while slowly breathing in and out. Change hand positions and repeat on the other side.

7 Place your hands back on your diaphragm (see second photograph, step 1) and concentrate on the movement of your breath inside your body.

Note: You will probably find at this point that it feels good to breathe in and out freely a few times to get ready for the next experience of breathing.

Become aware of your breathing. . .2

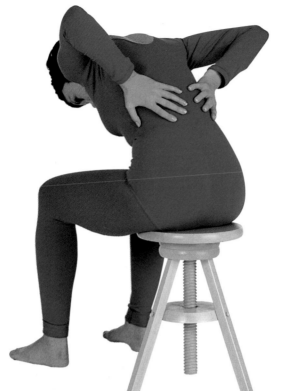

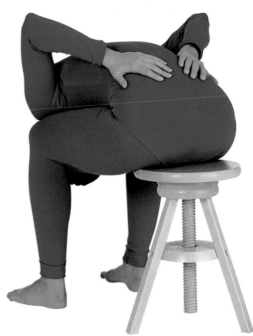

▲

1 Still sitting in the King's
position, place your legs about
hip-width apart and parallel to
each other. Bend your trunk slightly
forward and breathe in and out
twice, then place your hands on
the wall of the diaphragm at the
back with fingertips touching at
the spine. Now exhale and move
your palms over this part as you
did on the abdominal area in the
previous exercise (steps 2 to 3).

▲

2 When breathing on impulse,
or visualizing the movement of
air in your body, rest your trunk on
your thighs and follow the flow of
air along your spine. Sit up slowly
and breathe once more on
impulse. When you are
concentrating on the inner
movement of your breath you can
increase or decrease the flow but,
at this stage, inhaling and exhaling
deeply four times is enough.

Note: If you have someone with you who can place his or her hands on
your ribcage at the back, you will find it easier to feel the movements of
breath in your body. On your own you may need to repeat the exercise
frequently until you are sure you can follow your breath. If you can get your
hands high on the ribcage there should be no problem. There are a couple
of tricks to try: on a chair you can brace your ribcage against the back so
you get the necessary resistance; on a stool use a towel (held as if drying
yourself after a shower or bath) to help you feel the movement clearly.

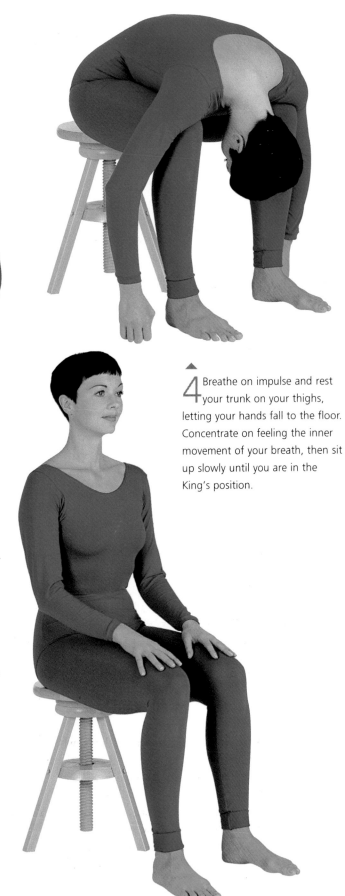

3 Sitting upright, place one hand palm down over your shoulder and resting on the spine. Bring your other arm round the side of your body, palm facing out. Inhale and exhale calmly and try to feel the movement of air. Repeat in the other direction. ▼

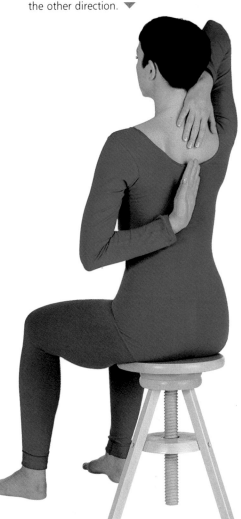

4 Breathe on impulse and rest your trunk on your thighs, letting your hands fall to the floor. Concentrate on feeling the inner movement of your breath, then sit up slowly until you are in the King's position.

5 Breathe freely. Now consider ▶ the depth of your awareness. Did you feel your breath in all areas of the body during this and the previous sequence? After a rest, repeat the exercise for those parts where you had difficulty following the movement.

Be at home with yourself

Imagine your body is a house and that it has elastic walls. By using your breath effectively you can expand the space inside, moving the oxygen-rich air so it freshens all parts of the body. This is the powerful fuel of health.

You will have felt some of the elasticity of your inner "walls" when doing the first exercise on pp. 38–41. Now you need to raise your awareness further by finding out how the breathing areas differ. Refresh your memory by looking at the information on pp. 16–17. The four breathing areas shown there all influence each other because of the complex interplay of muscles which connect them with each other and other parts of the body.

You will come across references to the breathing areas throughout the exercises in this part. The sequences within each exercise are designed to enable you to do more as your breathing becomes more proficient. After a while, when an exercise refers to a particular breathing area you will know from practice where in the body you should feel the movement of air. At the beginning however you may not find it easy to be precise. In the abdominal area, for instance, you may not be able to distinguish between breathing areas 1 and 2. Do not force it – just let the air flow.

You will find that the exercises make you take up positions which favour one or other of the breathing areas, and by following a daily routine your perception of them will increase.

So think of your "house". For stability you have foundations. Structure and support comes from the skeleton and the partitions are elastic. Here you learn to look inside this home – which is responsible for how you feel – and to know it well.

Home start

This is a 20-minute exercise with four sequences to increase your awareness of breathing areas 1 to 4. The aim is to make you more alert, improve the way you sit and encourage greater mobility of pelvis and diaphragm.

The sitting bones. . .1 ▶

1 Sit in the King's position ▶ (p. 25) with soles flat on the floor. Place one hand on the abdomen, the other on the lumbar region. Now move around on your buttocks, forward and backward, from left to right, slowly then quickly. You will feel the bones under your buttocks – these are your sitting bones, which are referred to constantly throughout the exercises. Sitting on your sitting bones gives you stability and balance.

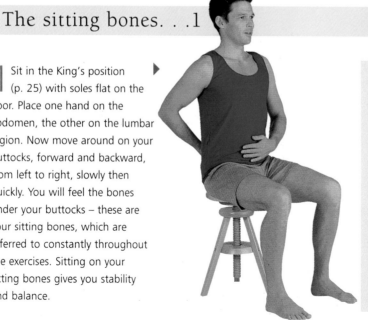

Well aired

You will find that some breathing areas are easier to feel than others when you begin breath training. But you become aware of them all once you are breathing consciously and the rhythm becomes more balanced. The whole of your "house" will then be well aired, with no part polluted by stale, unmoving air.

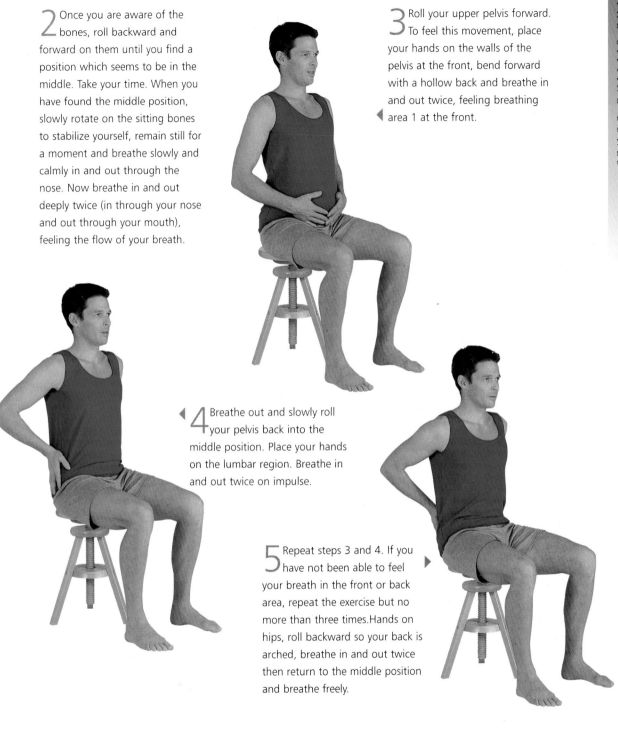

2 Once you are aware of the bones, roll backward and forward on them until you find a position which seems to be in the middle. Take your time. When you have found the middle position, slowly rotate on the sitting bones to stabilize yourself, remain still for a moment and breathe slowly and calmly in and out through the nose. Now breathe in and out deeply twice (in through your nose and out through your mouth), feeling the flow of your breath.

3 Roll your upper pelvis forward. To feel this movement, place your hands on the walls of the pelvis at the front, bend forward with a hollow back and breathe in and out twice, feeling breathing area 1 at the front.

4 Breathe out and slowly roll your pelvis back into the middle position. Place your hands on the lumbar region. Breathe in and out twice on impulse.

5 Repeat steps 3 and 4. If you have not been able to feel your breath in the front or back area, repeat the exercise but no more than three times. Hands on hips, roll backward so your back is arched, breathe in and out twice then return to the middle position and breathe freely.

Note: If your feet are the foundations of your house, the sitting bones and pelvis are the floorboards of the first floor. The floorboards are solid and can support great weight. The sitting bones provide stability while the pelvis carries the weight.

The sitting bones. . .2

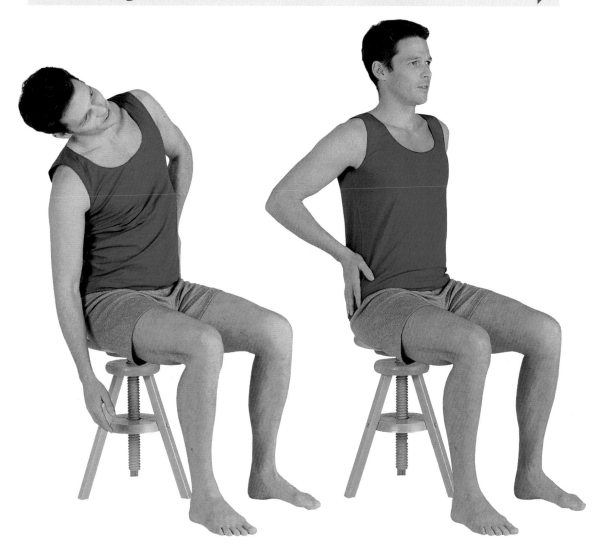

1 Still sitting in the middle position, let your right arm drop down and place your left hand on your side. Bend to the right until you feel a slight pull in breathing area 2 on your left. The weight of your body should be on your left leg. Apply slight pressure with the right foot to steady yourself. Hold this position while breathing in and out twice. You will be feel your breath clearly in breathing area 2 on the left.

2 Move back to the middle position and breathe on impulse. Now repeat step 1 on your left side. Concentrate on "looking into" your breathing areas. You will become more and more aware of them throughout your breath training programme.

3 Move back to the middle position, with your weight carried equally by your buttocks and your "house" (your trunk) resting on the biggest bone of your body, the pelvis. Become aware of your posture: you are sitting straight, erect – looking most regal. You are now back in the King's position.

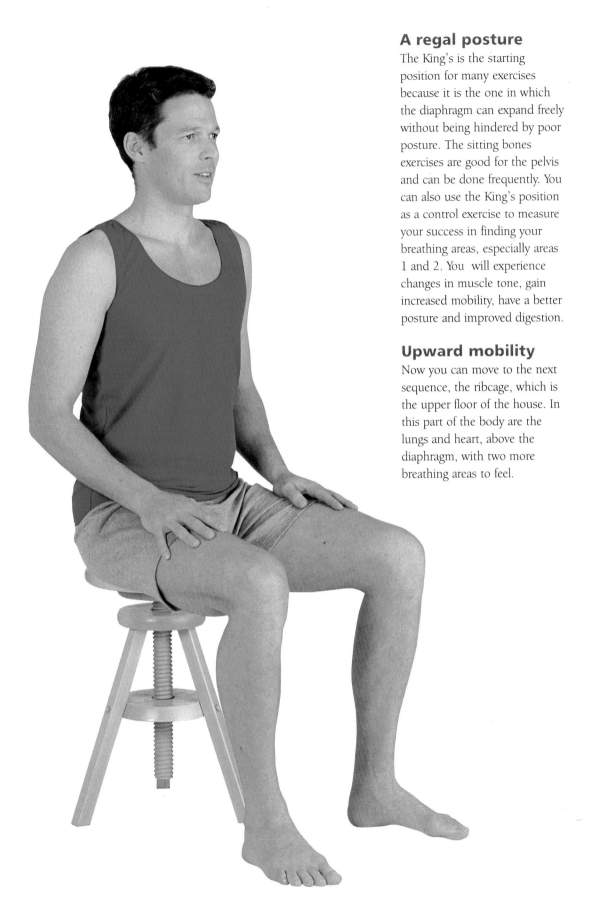

A regal posture

The King's is the starting position for many exercises because it is the one in which the diaphragm can expand freely without being hindered by poor posture. The sitting bones exercises are good for the pelvis and can be done frequently. You can also use the King's position as a control exercise to measure your success in finding your breathing areas, especially areas 1 and 2. You will experience changes in muscle tone, gain increased mobility, have a better posture and improved digestion.

Upward mobility

Now you can move to the next sequence, the ribcage, which is the upper floor of the house. In this part of the body are the lungs and heart, above the diaphragm, with two more breathing areas to feel.

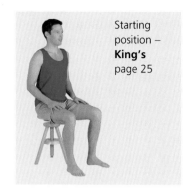

Starting
position –
King's
page 25

Ribs and diaphragm. . . .1

1 Place your hands firmly on the
side walls of your ribcage.
Spread your palms so they cover a
large part of your chest. Breathe
freely in and out. ▶

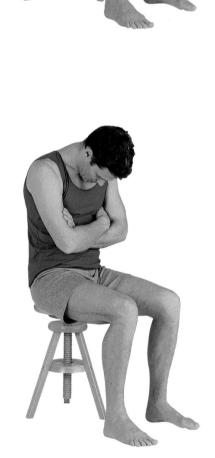

2 Keeping the weight on your
sitting bones, concentrate on
your rib cage. Breathe out and
move your chest away from the
middle, breathe in and move it
back. Move it twice in each
direction, to the right, left, front
and back, then breathe freely. If
the movement did not feel easy,
repeat this step.

3 Each time you breathe out
rotate your chest two to three
times. If when you exhale you
hear a low moan, breathe two to
three times. Most of your body
weight is still carried by the pelvis.
Move back to the middle position
and breathe freely.

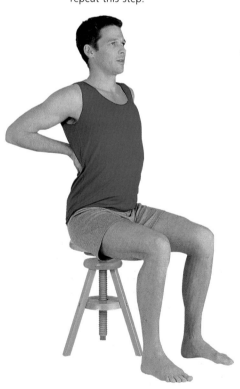

◀ 4 Rest your hands on your back
on the wall of the diaphragm.
Move your chest forward (the
weight resting on the pelvis also
shifts a little). Breathe twice on
impulse in this position. You
should now be able to feel
breathing area 3. Drop your hands
to your sides, move back to the
middle position and breathe freely.

5 Cross your arms in front of ▶
you, bending the upper part
of your back, including your
head, forward. You can feel the air
in breathing area 3 when you
breathe in and out twice. Uncross
your arms, move back to the
middle position and breathe freely.

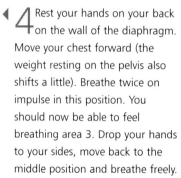

Ribs and diaphragm. . .2

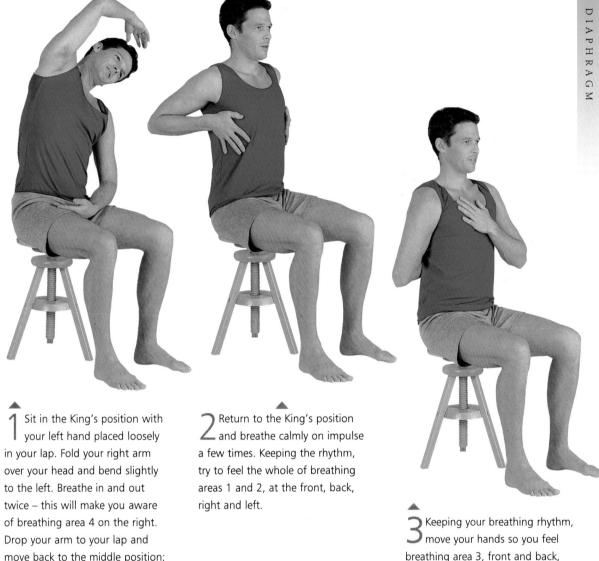

▲
1 Sit in the King's position with your left hand placed loosely in your lap. Fold your right arm over your head and bend slightly to the left. Breathe in and out twice – this will make you aware of breathing area 4 on the right. Drop your arm to your lap and move back to the middle position; breathe on impulse. Repeat, folding your left arm over your head and bending to the right.

▲
2 Return to the King's position and breathe calmly on impulse a few times. Keeping the rhythm, try to feel the whole of breathing areas 1 and 2, at the front, back, right and left.

▲
3 Keeping your breathing rhythm, move your hands so you feel breathing area 3, front and back, and breathing area 4, left and right. The lungs are in these areas.

Moving on: Once you are really confident about the sitting position and breathing areas, you can progress to the following exercises which have names that describe the movements involved – for example, you will move like a pendulum swings, be as lithe as a cat or as soft as a cloud. When you feel you have mastered one, move on to the next. With continuous exercise and an established daily routine, the pace and power of your breathing will improve enormously and you can then make up your own programme.

The Pendulum

Duration: 10–15 minutes.

Aim: To be aware of the rhythm and pace of your breathing, to change and modify it.

Mental attitude:
To move into an ever increasing state of well-being, guided by the rhythm of your breath.

Positive side-effects:
Stretching and straightening the body enables you to remain seated or standing for a long time.

Ultimate effect: Balance and increased energy.

Your breath has the same movements as a pendulum in this exercise. In the six sequences you should always keep the same rhythm – breathe out … pause … breathe in. This rhythm is only interrupted by a natural impulse to take a deep breath – or heave a sigh – which releases tension and makes you more alert so you breathe freely. After this, your breathing returns to the rhythmic movements of the pendulum.

By surrendering to this regular rhythm and following the flow of air, your whole body is engaged in the movement of your breath. How slowly or quickly you breathe is influenced by impulses from outside and inside the body and can change, consciously or unconsciously.

This exercise allows you to speed up or slow down your breathing, which can be useful in a variety of situations. The swinging movement of your body will be both energizing and improve your balance.

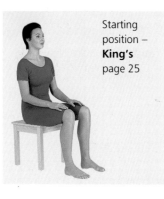

Starting position –
King's
page 25

Getting into the swing. . .1 ▶

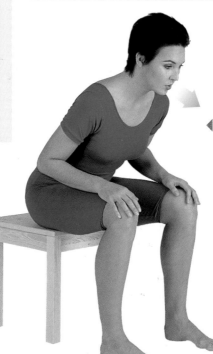

1 Focus on something in front of you on the floor. Imagine a camera inside you moving up and down filming your breath.

2 Breathe out gently with your lips slightly pursed (as if whistling), swinging slightly forward. Keep your trunk stretched and move your hips not the spine.

3 Pause by relaxing your lips, tongue and jaws, then close your lips lightly and inhale through your nose.

4 As you breathe out, be aware of your body's physical centre, 2–3 cm (1–1½ in) below the navel. On the next in-breath swing back to the upright position. ▼

5 Continue in this way, being aware of the pendulum-like rhythm of your breath. Inhaling and exhaling should take the same amount of time.

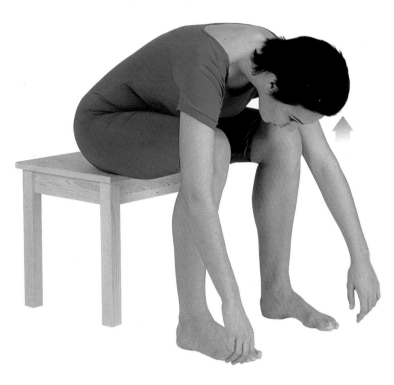

Suggestion for the day

A few times during the day stop whatever you are doing and tune in to your spiritual self, listening to the rhythm of your breathing. Check whether your physical and mental movements differ from your breathing rhythm. Concentrate on swinging them all back into balance.

6 When body and breath are in the same swinging rhythm expand the movement, swinging further and further forward but only until you become aware of your body's centre of gravity. Support yourself with a little foot pressure if necessary.

7 Reduce the swing gradually until you return to the King's position. Breathe on impulse.

Getting into the swing. . .2 ▶

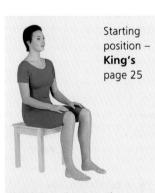

Starting position – **King's** page 25

Your arms become the pendulum which swings in semicircles over your head and out to the front.

1 Breathe in, slightly bending your trunk forward and turning your head to the right. Breathe out as you swing your left arm over your head in a semicircle to the right. ▶

2 Inhale and swing your left arm to the front across the knees in a semicircle back to the left side. Straighten up with arms by your sides and breathe out. Inhale at the height of the pendulum movement.

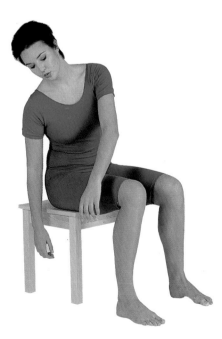

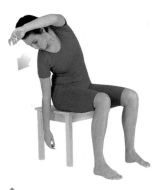
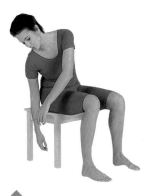
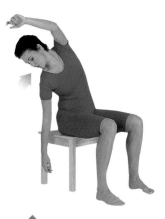

3 Keeping the rhythm of your breathing, repeat step 2 but from right to left. Continue like this until you have successfully performed several small semicircles to the right and left, breathing deeply.

4 Now let the rhythm of your breath increase as you make increasingly large semicircles, stretching high over your head and reaching wide in front so your trunk rests on your thighs as your arm swings back to the starting point.

5 Continue to swing rhythmically as you gradually reduce the size of the semicircles. Imagine the pendulum of a grandfather clock slowly coming to a halt. Rest.

Time to pause

Always pause to take some deep breaths during these movements, especially when the pendulum makes larger circles. You need to increase the length of the pauses before

you inhale Try not to breathe in too much air, allowing it.to flow in only when you perform the last movement of the swinging pendulum. This gives you more time to exhale and to get rid of air you don't need.

Getting into the swing. . .3

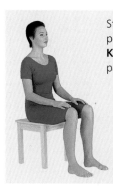

Starting position – **King's** page 25

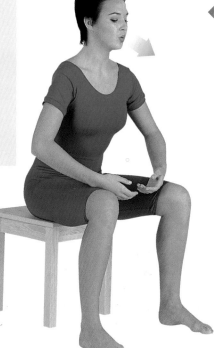

1 Sit with your wrists resting lightly above your knees. Relax your shoulders and stretch your neck. When you are aware of the rhythm of your breath heave a sigh, exhale and swing forward to place your weight firmly on your legs and feet. Pause, let go of the air.

2 Relax your lips, tongue and face muscles, putting out your tongue occasionally to open up the pharynx (a good exercise if you have a throat infection). Inhale and swing back to the starting position. Repeat up to five times.

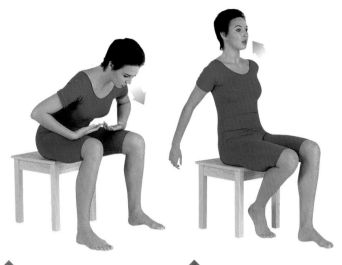

3 Breathe out on a sigh and swing forward; pause in this position and put out your tongue. Breathe in as you close your mouth and swing back. Then carry on breathing in your normal rhythm.

4 Move to the edge of the seat with your arms hanging loose. Place your left foot flat on the floor and your right foot under the seat, resting on the toes. On exhaling swing your trunk forward; swing back when inhaling. Move further and further forward, shifting your body's weight on to your left foot as you swing.

Move ahead

The emphasis in this part of the exercise is on the forward movement. When you breathe in you do not straighten up completely but remain slightly bent forward to shift the weight a little further back and on to the right foot. Breathing out gives you impetus but you breathe in rapidly. The more you intensify this, the stronger the breathing reflex becomes. You can let go quickly when you pause and breathe in more rapidly after the pause. In order not to hinder this vitalizing process, inhale and exhale through your mouth when the movements increase.

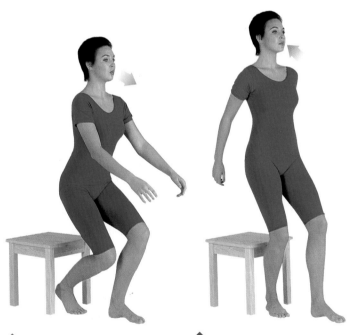

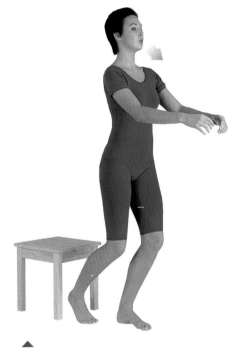

5 With your weight increasingly on your left foot your body is lifted off the seat on a forward swing. Shift the weight back to the right foot again when you breathe in and swing back.

6 Swing from one foot to the other, switching your body weight from one to the other, and gradually stretching your trunk until you are upright.

7 With your knees bent – to trigger breathing on impulse – swing forward and backward a few times. Decrease the movement gradually, coming to rest with your weight on both legs.

Rhythm and movement . . . 1

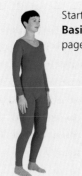

Starting position –
Basic
page 20

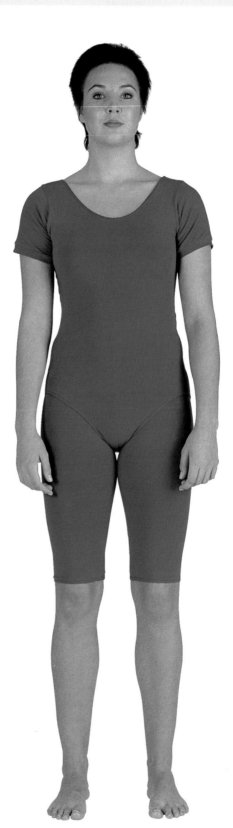

1 Rest your weight on your heels, the balls of your feet, the outer edges of your soles and your big toes. Keep feet flat, your shoulders loose and your body straight. All your joints should be open, not locked.

2 Focus on something on the floor in front of you, then concentrate on the movement of your breath. Inhale and exhale without guiding your breath, but become aware of movement and rhythm. Watch how the air flows into all breathing areas and flows out again. Then stop watching and feel what else is happening to you and your body.

3 If your nose, mouth, diaphragm and chest are open to the movement of air, you will notice your body is swinging slightly – like a slow pendulum.

4 When you stop focusing carry on swinging gently for a little while. Keep one eye on what is happening inside your body and look around you with the other.

Balancing tension

The fact that you are breathing means that your body is constantly moving. If you allow it to happen, the movement balances tensions by keeping them in check. When you swing you gather strength which is transmitted to the muscles through the open joints. You can literally swing into the right posture and rebalance yourself.

Rhythm and movement. . . 2

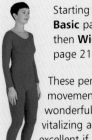

Starting position – **Basic** page 20, then **Wide-hipped** page 21

These pendulum movements are wonderfully vitalizing and are excellent if you are tense or lack energy. But only attempt them if you have mastered the exercises on pp. 48–52 and feel comfortable doing them.

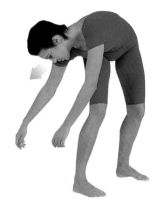

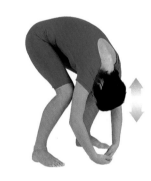

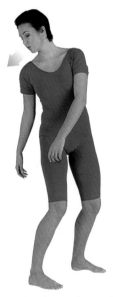

1 Stand with your knees slightly bent. Breathe out and let your left arm swing to your right; breathe in and let it swing back to the left. Your trunk follows the direction of the arm movement.

2 Repeat a few times with both arms until you can really feel them swing and your body is rotating round its centre. Keep your feet flat – the wider you swing the more your knees bend.

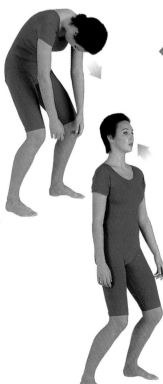

3 To increase the intensity of the movement swing the arms low at your sides to pull the trunk forward. Slowly let go and swing deep to your right while exhaling; deep to your left when inhaling. Ensure your feet remain flat and your legs provide stability.

4 Vary the swinging with other movements – straightening up and slightly crouching. Breathing out forcefully rids the lungs of air and triggers the impulse to inhale which allows air to flow in and creates energy.

5 To calm down, make only small but well-balanced movements and always be aware of your legs supporting your body weight. Listen to the rhythm of your breath until you are completely calm and still.

6 With knees bent, breathe out and roll down the vertebrae from your neck to the base of the spine. Do it at a pace that feels comfortable; breathing out as you roll and stopping to breathe in if it feels natural. Return gradually to the Wide-hipped position.

Control note

If you feel dizzy at any time during this sequence, the Regaining control exercise (p. 54) will stabilize your circulation. It is also ideal when you feel you are about to lose your temper.

Regaining control

If you feel dizzy or about to lose your temper, this is a simple exercise which will stabilize your circulation and settle you down.

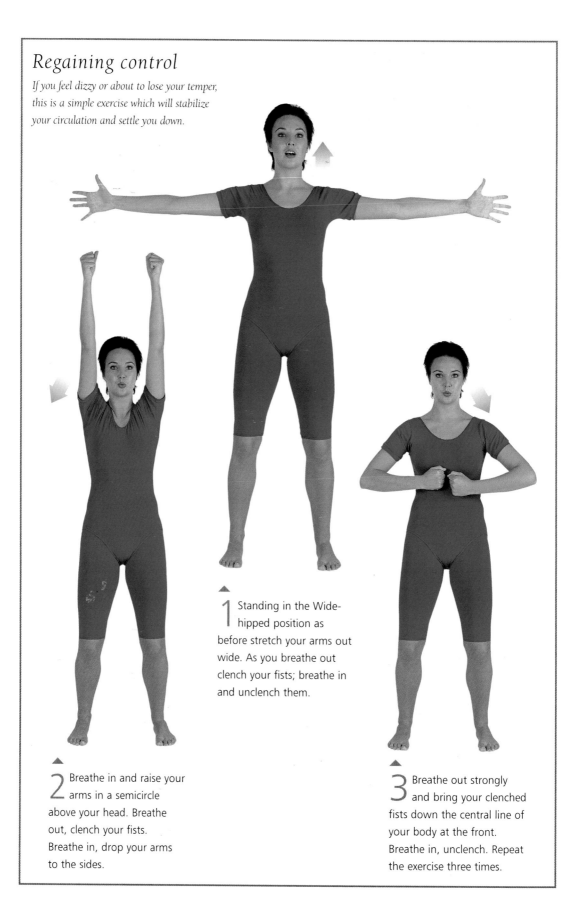

1 Standing in the Wide-hipped position as before stretch your arms out wide. As you breathe out clench your fists; breathe in and unclench them.

2 Breathe in and raise your arms in a semicircle above your head. Breathe out, clench your fists. Breathe in, drop your arms to the sides.

3 Breathe out strongly and bring your clenched fists down the central line of your body at the front. Breathe in, unclench. Repeat the exercise three times.

Rhythm and movement. . . 3

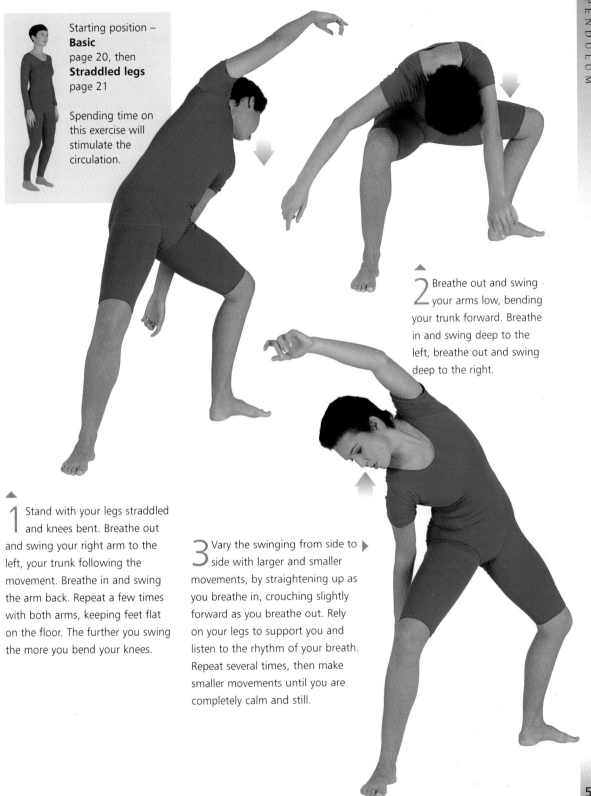

Starting position –
Basic
page 20, then
Straddled legs
page 21

Spending time on
this exercise will
stimulate the
circulation.

2 Breathe out and swing
your arms low, bending
your trunk forward. Breathe
in and swing deep to the
left, breathe out and swing
deep to the right.

1 Stand with your legs straddled
and knees bent. Breathe out
and swing your right arm to the
left, your trunk following the
movement. Breathe in and swing
the arm back. Repeat a few times
with both arms, keeping feet flat
on the floor. The further you swing
the more you bend your knees.

3 Vary the swinging from side to
side with larger and smaller
movements, by straightening up as
you breathe in, crouching slightly
forward as you breathe out. Rely
on your legs to support you and
listen to the rhythm of your breath.
Repeat several times, then make
smaller movements until you are
completely calm and still.

The Cradle

Duration: 15 minutes.

Aim: To activate breathing area 1 and release tension in the back (spine, muscles and diaphragm).

Mental attitude:
Relaxed, as if lying in a cradle which gently starts to rock.

Positive side-effects:
Balancing the tension in the back muscles; balancing and in some cases correcting the posture of the spine.

Ultimate effect:
Deep effective breathing in breathing area 1; strengthening leg, stomach and back muscles.

This exercise has four sequences and is recommended in times of stress when you are out of touch with your calm inner self. Healthy breathing enables air to move freely throughout your body. When the breath permeates the muscles, it is not just the elastic walls that must be able to give and expand. Many parts of the skeleton must be able to do so too. With the help of the Cradle actions, small irregularities of the spine can be corrected. They can also ease and heal imbalances of breathing and posture, and relieve uncomfortable back muscles which have become unhealthy through tension. You can relax the parts of the back under the greatest strain, especially the area around the lumbar spine, and gain calm, uninterrupted breathing.

Starting position –
The dune
page 28

Place the palms of your hands on your abdomen between your chestbone and pubic bone. Breathe out, feeling your abdomen fall. This is a passive kind of sinking; do not force it. Pause and release all tension before the next in-breath which should reach breathing area 1.

Rocking and rolling. . .1 ▶

1 You should feel the sacrum (the lowest part of the spine) touching the floor. Activate the sacrum by gently rolling from one side to the other. Supporting yourself on your forearms and feet, lift your pelvis and make circling movements, to the left then the right. Pause. Breathe on impulse. Feel your weight and sacrum pressing on the floor.

Suggestion for the day

In your thoughts, move up and down your spine several times a day. Gently rock it with every breath you take. Use your hands to feel breathing area 1.

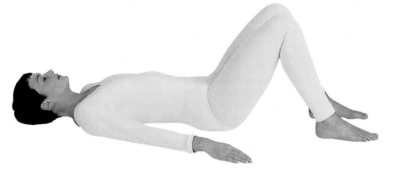

2 Place your arms by your sides slightly away from your body. Breathe evenly and become aware of its rhythm. Each time you exhale support your weight with the right, then with the left, leg. Do not force anything – just be able to feel your pelvis and lower back on the floor.

3 Breathe in while you release the pressure of one foot after the other, rocking your legs gently and consistently from side to side. Do this about five times until the movements and the rhythm of your breath harmonize, then breathe deeply. Imagine your breath is "trickling" into the breathing area like a warm stream.

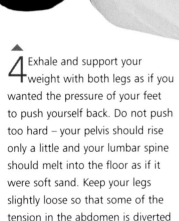

4 Exhale and support your weight with both legs as if you wanted the pressure of your feet to push yourself back. Do not push too hard – your pelvis should rise only a little and your lumbar spine should melt into the floor as if it were soft sand. Keep your legs slightly loose so that some of the tension in the abdomen is diverted to them for stability.

5 Repeat steps 1 to 4 three to five times; then rest and breathe on impulse. Imagine you are in a large and beautiful room flooded with sunlight.

Suggestion for the evening

If you feel the need to relax, lie in the Dune position, on the floor or sofa. Now breathe calmly and regularly, feeling the lumbar spine and abdomen sinking gradually into the carpet or cushions.

Releasing energy

Activating the sacrum by rocking and rolling releases energy that is buried deep down. It also gives mobility to the area where the sacrum meets the lumbar spine, making it easier to shift the weight to the stronger pelvis. The tension is diverted, the upper breathing areas are freed and the lower ones strengthened.

Rocking and rolling. . .2

1 Support yourself by equal foot pressure. Breathe out and roll the pelvis off the floor, then back on to it. Pause and release all tension, then breathe in. Now roll the lumbar spine vertebra by vertebra on one out-breath. Pause and breathe in, then roll back.

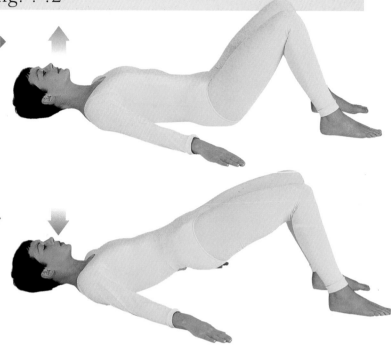

2 Move on to rolling the thoracic spine in the same way, vertebra by vertebra, to shoulder level. Support your weight on your legs and pelvis, with your shoulders and arms resting passively. If you cannot do this smoothly, rest and rock to and fro a few times – breathe in, apply foot pressure to one leg, roll up three or four vertebrae, roll back.

Slowly does it

Do this exercise in small doses – at first roll two or three of the vertebrae of your lumbar spine, building up to all five. Guide your breath when exhaling (making sounds like sh, s, f or mm) to ensure your movements are slow and the breathing area is gradually opened up. Keep your abdomen soft.

3 To strengthen your breathing capacity even further try to roll up and back down again on one out-breath. Do this only when you feel really comfortable with the movement. Your breath will become even stronger the longer you take to exhale.

Rocking and rolling. . . 3

Note: Only attempt this sequence if you have no problems with your spine. The aim is to strengthen and shape the muscles in the legs and buttocks.

1 Lie on your back and stretch yourself, then roll on to your stomach. Place your hands under your forehead.

2 Breathe out as you gently press your pubic bone to the floor, at the same time stretching your right leg away from your

body to the side. Lift the heel until you can feel the muscles of the leg and buttocks tensing a little.

3 Guide your breath out and let go of the tension when you inhale. Tension should be restricted to the leg and buttocks to ensure air can flow into breathing area 1.

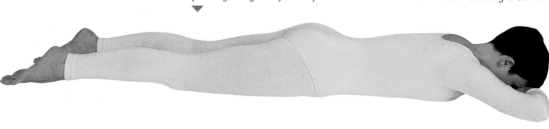

Having problems?

The rocking and rolling movements of the Cradle exercise should be smooth and even – and it may take you some time to achieve this. Repeat the first two sequences until you feel confident that you can feel the movement of your breath inside you. After completing Rocking and rolling 2, release the tension in the pelvis by shifting your body weight to your buttocks. Finally, breathe deeply, feeling breathing area 1 flooding with air.

4 Stretch your leg as step 2 twice, then hold it off the floor and inhale. Guide your breath out while lowering your leg slowly – do not let it fall as this will defeat the purpose. ▼

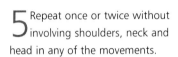

5 Repeat once or twice without involving shoulders, neck and head in any of the movements.

6 Repeat steps 2 to 5, this time using your left leg.

7 Pause and breathe deeply. Exhale and lift one leg off the floor three times without resting in between, then repeat with your other leg. Gradually become aware of the movement of your breath in breathing area 1 (especially at the back). Stretch ◀ your arms loosely in front of you.

8 Lift your right leg upward from your body, breathe out and stretch your raised left arm. Inhale, lift arm and leg a little higher, then exhale and slowly lower them. ▶

9 Repeat twice, each time trying to lift your arm and leg a little higher. Enjoy the tension you feel diagonally across your back, from heel to fingertips, but stop immediately if it hurts. You should feel your breath in breathing area 1 and slight tension in your neck.

10 Breathe in and place your hands under your forehead. Breathe out, pressing your pubic bone to the floor and lifting both legs upward. With your chest against the floor, feel the tension in your legs and buttocks. Slowly lower your legs. ▼

11 Repeat steps 8–10 using the opposite arm and leg. If you apply all your concentration to this sequence you should only have to repeat it once, then relax and breathe deeply.

Note: When you first do this sequence, finish at step 11 and move on to Rocking and rolling 4 (p. 61). After a few sessions you should be able to return to this section and continue with steps 12 to 16 (p. 60).

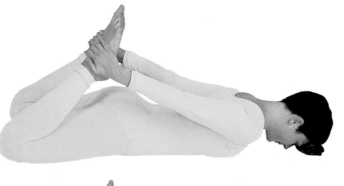

12 Use a pad to cushion your forehead. Reach back with both arms to hold your insteps with your hands. Each time you exhale pull your left, then your right, heel on to your thigh. Do this five times with each leg. If you feel too much tension in your thighs pause before each pull.

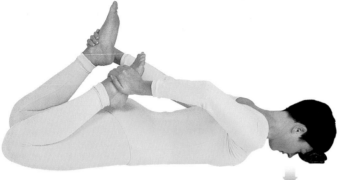

13 After a short rest take hold of your insteps again. Breathe out and pull each leg away from your body. This will lift your shoulders and head slightly. Do this two to three times.

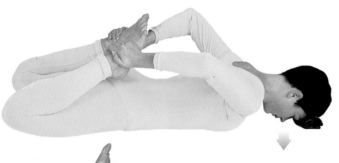

14 Lift legs, pelvis, shoulders and head and start rocking yourself gently, breathing out as you rock forward and in as you rock backward. If you can do this with ease you have exercised your abdomen as well, increasing the volume of breath.

15 Keeping the rhythm of rocking and breathing (in, backward; out, forward) increase the speed gradually until you are swinging, then slow down again to rocking movements.

16 Take your hands off your feet and rest your trunk on the floor. Breathe on impulse. Place your hands under your forehead and feel the flow of your breath everywhere in your body. ▼

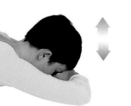

Rocking and rolling. . .4

Starting position –
The package
page 29

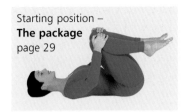

1 Rest your shoulders and head comfortably on the floor. Breathe out rapidly and strongly as you pull both knees to your chest, moving your elbows out to the side to keep your shoulders and neck passive. ▼

2 Breathe in as you move your knees back to their original position. Repeat at least five times. Now pull your knees alternately up to your chest, five times with each, breathing out rapidly and strongly. The lumbar spine will become round and soft, like a bow. Breathe on impulse. ▼

3 Hold right knee with both hands and pull it to your chest. Stretch the left leg up, but do not tense it. By slightly moving your upstretched leg start rocking, exhaling as you rock forward and inhaling as you rock backward. ▼

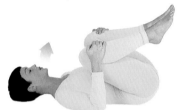

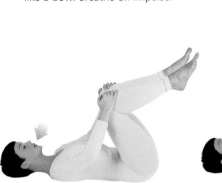

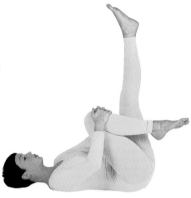

4 Keep your head aligned with your spine and slightly bent forward. Rock and swing until you are in a sitting position (it will happen automatically after rocking to and fro three to five times). ▼

5 Once you are sitting, try to round your spine while breathing out, then inhale and roll gently backward. Give yourself a push and instantly sit up again. Roll back up to five times and instantly swing forward again with every out-breath. ▼

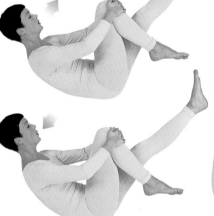

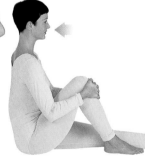

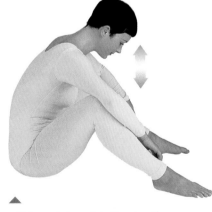

6 Repeat steps 3 to 5, using the other leg. Finish the sequence with feet on the floor, head and arms relaxed. Breathe on impulse.

The Cat

Duration: 15 minutes.

Aim: To achieve flexibility of the trunk; to stretch gently and open up breathing areas 2 and 4.

Mental attitude:
I have become as lithe as a cat.

Positive side-effects:
Increased mobility and flexibility; counter-balancing scoliosis (lateral curvature of the spine).

Ultimate effect:
Strengthening legs, buttocks, pelvis and the back muscles.

You only have to watch a cat move to appreciate its sinuous and free style. There is no tension, just a smooth harmony and elegant action as the breath moves through the body without meeting any resistance. Think of this in relation to yourself. Breathing freely relieves you of unnecessary tension. When you are only doing light work the muscles involved get the chance to exercise their power while others are free from tension.

In the five sequences of this exercise you will find how to use your body's power and energy more economically so your body can endure more and keep going for longer. You will be able to rest and relax between different activities yet remain alert and ready to act – just as a cat is watchful and moves swiftly to play. When your breath is relaxed and muscle tension eased they can regenerate; should you need more energy, they react quickly and provide stimulation. Relaxed is not passive. It's powerful.

Shoulder lift

This is an excellent exercise for anyone whose shoulders tend to sag or whose back is rounded.

1 On your knees with your buttocks raised, breathe out and stretch your left arm out in front of you, turning your head toward your right arm. You should feel comfortable, as if leisurely stretching yourself. Keep your back soft and elastic.

2 Breathing freely, continue in this way stretching each arm alternately while turning your head in the opposite direction. Ensure the buttocks remain behind your knees to create the necessary counter-pull between the arms, shoulders and pelvis at the back.

3 Carry on stretching your arms with your armpits gradually getting closer to the floor. Then, with both arms outstretched in front, take two deep breaths. Inhale and roll yourself up, vertebra by vertebra, until you rest on your heels.

4 Breathe on impulse and feel whether the breathing areas have been opened up. Can you feel your breath in areas 3 and 4?

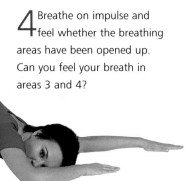

Stretch and strengthen. . . 1

Starting position –
The sphinx
page 23, then
Crouching
page 24

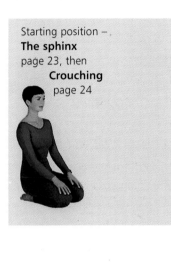

1 Kneel on your gym mat, sit back on your heels then crouch, placing your head on your hands in front of you. Breathe in and out three times, accompanying each out-breath with a sigh (like a cat's purr).

2 Breathing out with a sigh, let your arms glide forward along the mat until your buttocks lift off your heels and you can feel some stretching in your back and armpits. Make sure your buttocks remain behind your knees or your pelvis cannot support you. Your shoulders and arms should feel almost weightless. ▼

Suggestion for the day

Try and feel how flexible and mobile you are on the inside and outside of your body several times a day. Make round, soft movements to encourage flexibility.

3 Arms still forward, breathe in and pull yourself back, from the base of your spine until your buttocks rest on your heels.

4 Repeat the exercise five times. You do not have to reach your heels every time. Exhale and stretch yourself forward, inhale and pull yourself back again. Keep the arms relaxed, as your chestbone gradually gets closer to the floor. ▼

Stretch and strengthen. . .2

Starting position –
On all fours
page 24

Do this sequence very
slowly. Make sure you
breathe continuously and
that the movements of
your breath are regular.

1 Kneeling comfortably hollow
your back while breathing out.
Your head and neck will stretch
back, in line with your spine.
Breathe in, keeping this position. ▶

2 Breathe out and slowly roll
yourself back to the
horizontal, a movement carried out
by the lumbar spine – the
contraction in the abdominal
muscles is secondary. Breathe in
◀ again (while still horizontal).

3 Exhale while making your back
as round as you can. Do it very
slowly to balance possible spinal
irregularities and any tension in
your back. Stay in this position and
breathe in. Breathe out and roll
yourself back to the horizontal.
You should feel soft and relaxed,
if you don't, repeat this step. ▶

4 Still with your back horizontal,
breathe out and bend both
elbows outward. Exhale and make
your back hollow, stretching your
head and neck back and moving
your chin toward the floor. Breathe
in, letting yourself be pulled back,
from the base of the spine to the
◀ heels, then on to all fours with
your back arched.

5 Exhale while gently stretching
your back. Repeat hollowing
and rounding in this way three to
five times. You should feel a
wavelike movement the length of
your spine. ▼

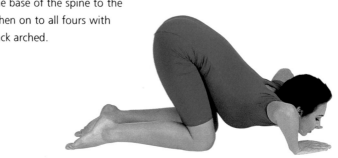

Stretch and strengthen. . . 3

1 On all fours, with your weight on your right knee, breathe out and slide your left leg away from you as your body comes to rest on your right heel. Your left groin is stretched. Breathe in, shift your weight to your right knee and draw the left leg back under you.

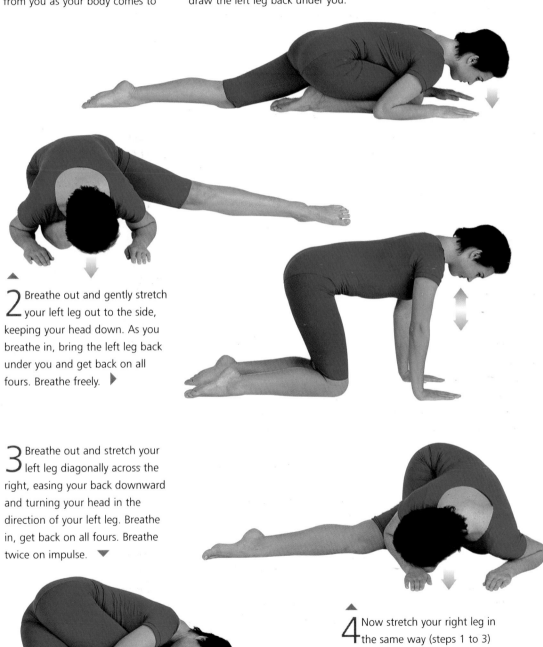

2 Breathe out and gently stretch your left leg out to the side, keeping your head down. As you breathe in, bring the left leg back under you and get back on all fours. Breathe freely. ▶

3 Breathe out and stretch your left leg diagonally across the right, easing your back downward and turning your head in the direction of your left leg. Breathe in, get back on all fours. Breathe twice on impulse. ▼

4 Now stretch your right leg in the same way (steps 1 to 3) to open up the pelvis and breathing areas 1 and 2. Make sure your movements are soft and regular. Repeat this sequence one to three times.

Side twist

1 On all fours, little by little move both hands in a curve toward your right knee. Only go as far as feels comfortable at first. Breathe out and move the hands a little more. Pause, breathe in and continue until your hands come to rest at the side of your knee. Move hands back to where they started from.

2 Now move your hands toward your left knee. Do it gently, little step by little step. Concentrate on your left side stretching – you should feel the breathing areas 2 and 4. Get back on to all fours and breathe in twice on impulse.

Note: If you find this short sequence difficult, do not force yourself to complete it. Remain in a position where you can feel the tension in your side. Take two to three deep breaths to release the tension – heave a big sigh if it makes you feel more comfortable and very slowly move your hands back to their original position.

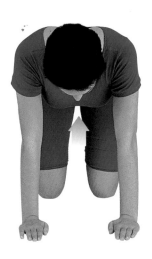
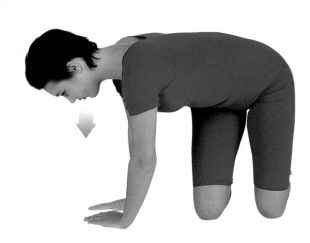

A longer stretch

A short sequence which challenges you to stretch and will strengthen your muscles. Do not attempt it if you have disc or back problems.

2 Breath out and try to stretch arm and leg a little more so you can feel your breath flowing from fingertips to toetips. Breathe out, get back on all fours. Repeat with right arm and left leg.

Note: You should be well-balanced. If you stretch your arm and leg too far you will feel unstable – but regular exercise will help you achieve balance.

1 Kneeling on all fours, make your left elbow touch your right knee (see step 3, opposite). Breathe out then stretch your left arm and right leg away from your body. Stretch so you feel the tension in fingertips and toes. Breathe in.

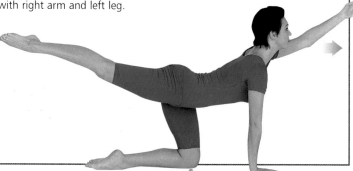

Stretch and strengthen. . .4

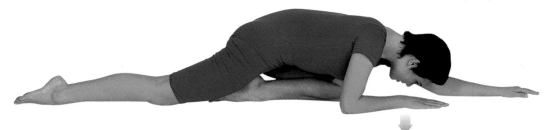

1 On all fours, breathe out and slide your left arm forward and right leg back, with your thigh – and thus your weight – coming to rest on your left heel.

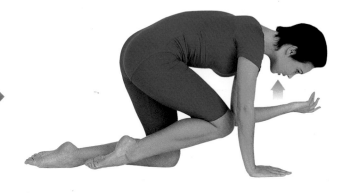

2 Breathe in, support yourself on your left knee, then come up again on to both knees, rounding your back gently.

Note: If you can't lower yourself and come up smoothly, start by sliding the leg and arm only a little way from the body and immediately coming up again.

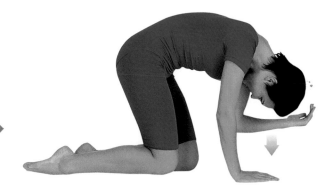

3 Exhale and bring your left elbow across to touch your raised right knee. Hold the position, pause, then inhale and return knee and hand to the floor.

4 Breathe out and stretch out your left arm and right leg, then pause, inhale and return both to the floor. Make all movements smooth. Repeat five to seven times, then do the same on the other side.

Stretch and strengthen. . . 5

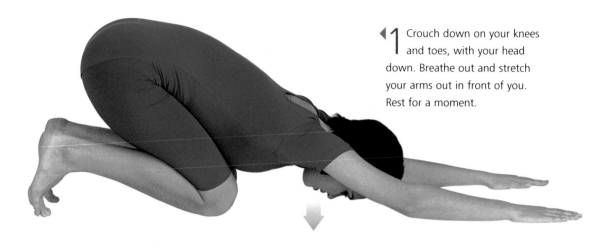

1 Crouch down on your knees and toes, with your head down. Breathe out and stretch your arms out in front of you. Rest for a moment.

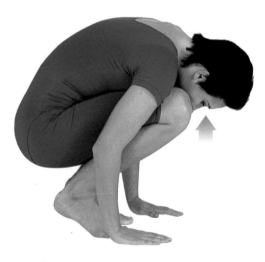

2 Inhale and pull your arms and trunk back until you are crouching like a cat. Breathe out, slowly raising your heels and resting on tiptoe with hands flat on the floor in front. Remain like this for a moment.

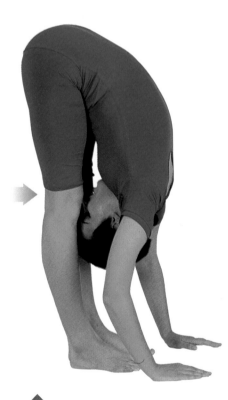

3 Breathe in and as you exhale gradually straighten your legs, keeping knees slightly bent and hands flat as your buttocks rise.

Suggestion for the day

Stop whatever you are doing and tune in to your spiritual self by listening to the rhythm of your breath. Do your physical and mental movements differ from your breathing rhythm? Concentrate on your breathing until you swing everything back into balance. On a stressful day you may need to do his several times, only for a few minutes.

Stretch to revive

Raising your arms above your head, reaching up as high as you can with your knees slightly bent, will revive tired muscles in the shoulders and neck. Bring your arms down to your side and roll your shoulders, first forward and then backward for an invigorating finishing touch.

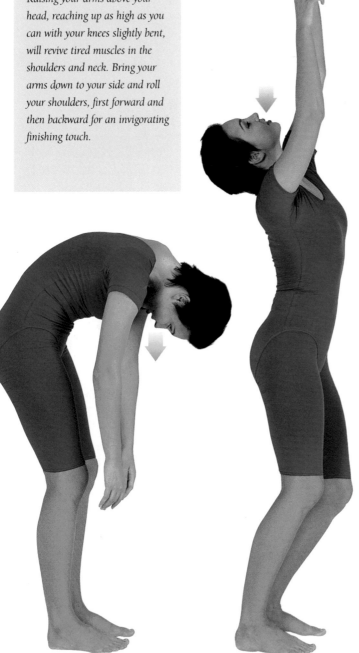

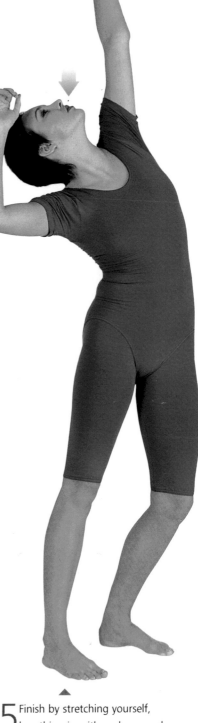

4 With one slow out-breath for each part of the spine roll upward, vertebra by vertebra. When upright, breathe deeply.

5 Finish by stretching yourself, breathing in with each upward reach, one arm at a time – stretch gracefully like a cat climbing a tree.

The Cloud

Duration: 15 minutes.

Aim:
To activate the diaphragm, the intercostal muscles and breathing areas 3 and 4.

Mental attitude:
Relaxed.

Positive side-effects:
Stimulation and cleansing of the lungs; a flexible and stimulated rib cage.

Ultimate effect:
Increase of a gentle but alert tension; self-confidence; clear perception of the movements of the diaphragm and breathing areas 3 and 4.

The diaphragm is a dome-shaped sheet of muscle which provides an efficient breathing system for the whole body. You can think of it as the "floor" of the thoracic cavity with lungs and heart above, or the "roof" of the abdominal cavity with all the other organs, like the liver and stomach, below. The way it works has a direct influence on all these organs. When you breathe in the diaphragm goes downward, providing space for the lungs to fill with air. When you exhale, the diaphragm goes up helping to push air out of the lungs. Elastic and flexible, it has "walls" which follow the shape of the ribcage, either side of the chestbone, across the back to the upper parts of the lumbar spine. You should treat this sensitive part of the body gently. Imagine you are leaning against something soft; this is how your breath expands in the middle of your body.

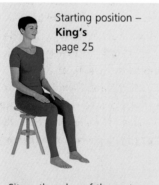

Starting position –
King's
page 25

Sit on the edge of the seat, in the middle of your sitting bones. You should be able to clearly feel breathing areas 1 and 2. If you can't, do one of the opening sequences first.

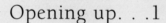

Opening up. . .1

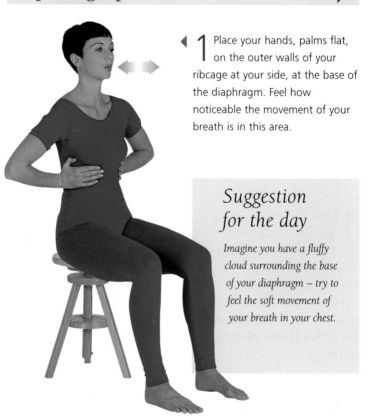

1 Place your hands, palms flat, on the outer walls of your ribcage at your side, at the base of the diaphragm. Feel how noticeable the movement of your breath is in this area.

Suggestion for the day

Imagine you have a fluffy cloud surrounding the base of your diaphragm – try to feel the soft movement of your breath in your chest.

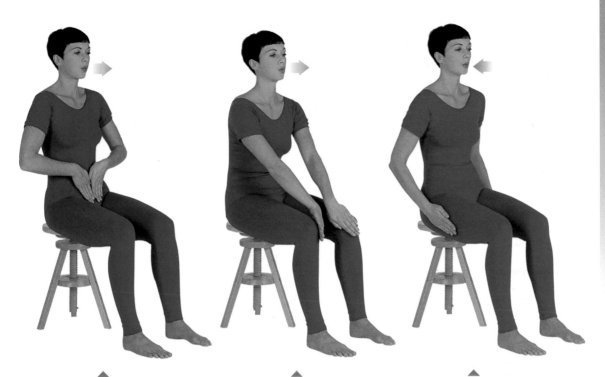

2 Breathe out and move your palms down to the middle of your body, then to your abdomen. Breathe in, moving palms across your pelvis and sides then back up to the chest. Feel the movement of your ribs under your palms. Repeat this circling, caressing movement up to five times, until you clearly feel your costal arches give under your palms. Each time increase pressure on the ribs.

3 Exhale and move your hands down along the inside of your thighs. Inhale and move them back to their original position along the outside of your thighs, the buttocks, the lumbar spine and the ribs on your lower back.

4 Continue making large circles, exhaling as you move your hands around your knees and to the outside of your thighs. Inhale as you move them back. Make your hands describe two large circles, then rest them by the side of your thighs and breathe deeply. You should now be able to feel breathing areas 1 and 2 clearly. If you can, move on to the sequence on page 72. If you can't, do Opening up 2 which starts below.

Opening up. . .2 ▶

1 Cross your arms, placing your ▶ palms on the walls of the ribcage so you have a good grip on your chest. Move your palms even further back, as far as possible. Your chest now should be resting in your arms. This activates and stimulates even the lowest and slackest parts of your lungs.

Note: You gain most from short exercises done often. Stop exercising as soon as you feel any discomfort. Breathe on impulse after each exercise.

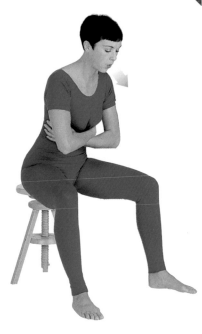

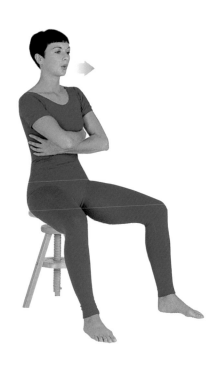

2 Breathe out strongly but freely and push the halves of your ribcage toward each other. Let go while breathing out; keep your arms crossed. Exhale again, bend slightly forward; remain bent and inhale. Breathe out again, bend forward further. After about five out-breaths your elbows will touch your knees. Take two deep breaths.

3 Exhale and pull yourself upright, keeping your arms crossed. Breathe in and on a slow out-breath guide your chest anti-clockwise in a semicircle to your left side, then back to the middle again. Breathe in, pause, breathe out and describe the same circle to the right side. Exhale, uncross your arms, rest.

Expand and accumulate. . . 1 ▶

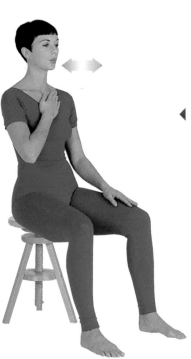

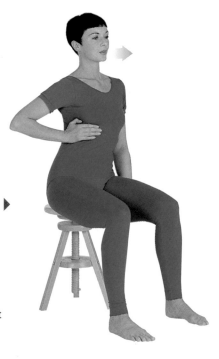

1 Breathe out, place your right palm on your left side, near the collarbone. Feel your breath sinking down your chest. Breathe in and lift your hand; breathe out and move your palm in stages toward your heart. With each in-breath change sides and hands. Continue until your breathing is calm and composed.

2 With your left arm hanging loosely, place your right hand on your right ribcage. Breathe out three times and little by little push your chest further and further to the left. Breathe out deeply a fourth time and push your chest even further. Breathe in, release hand pressure so the chest moves back to the middle. Repeat up to three times, then work on your left side in the same way.

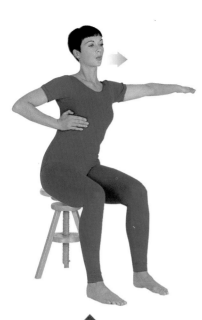

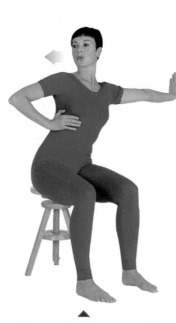

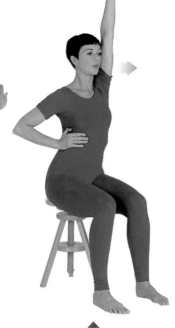

3 With your right hand on your ribcage stretch out your left arm with palm down. Repeat the movement of step 2, pushing your chest (and thus your trunk) on each out-breath, three times.

4 Turn your hand up – you will feel the tension in the wrist. Imagine yourself on a cluster of clouds pushing the clouds away. Breathe in and push your left hand away from your body while the right pushes your chest. Turn your head to the right, breathe out and relax your shoulders. Breathe in, then exhale and turn your outstretched palm down. Let your head flop. Inhale and release the hand pressure on your chest.

5 With your next out-breath stretch your left arm upward, palm up. Imagine your head is also trying to push the soft clouds up. Feel your spine stretching upward as you push your chest sideways.. Inhale, release pressure; exhale push the chest and stretch arm.

6 Finally, push the clouds away in front, palm up. Exercise your left side the same way, up to three times for each movement.

Expand and accumulate. . .2

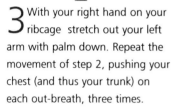

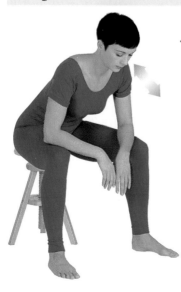

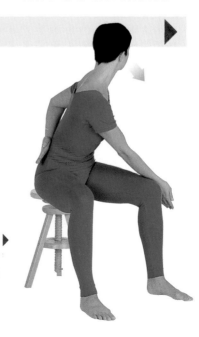

1 In the Seated coachman's position, rest and breathe freely. Breathe in and loosely stretch your right arm, palm outward, diagonally across your left leg. As you exhale, let your shoulders sag and place your left arm loosely on your back.

2 With every following out-breath turn your trunk further to the left and slide your right arm downward. Repeat three times.

73

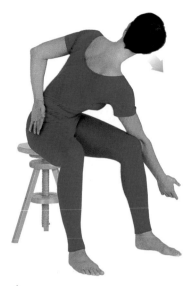 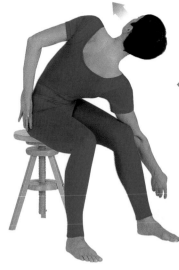

4 Breathe deeply and slowly get back into the original position. Before you start exercising in the other direction rest for a moment in the Seated coachman's position.

Note: When you have completed the exercise on both sides of the body rest again in the Seated coachman's position. Change to the King's position and pause a moment more. Sniff a little – as you might do when entering a room and trying to identify which familiar smells it holds – to make sure your ribcage and diaphragm are now more elastic.

3 Breathe out quickly and stretch each arm gently diagonally. Your trunk also turns further to the left. Your head is turned so that you are looking toward your left shoulder. Repeat this movement two to five times – you should feel comfortable doing it.

Expand and accumulate. . .3

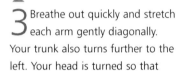 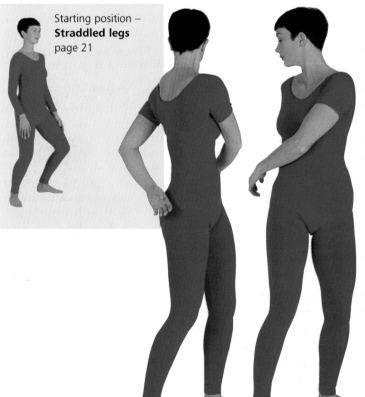

Starting position –
Straddled legs
page 21

1 Move to an area where you have enough space to stretch your arms in every direction. Start to twist to the right and the left, breathing out at each change of side. Your arms follow this movement, wrapping around your body and your head follows the arm swing in front.

2 The more you twist the more your arms wrap around your body. When you gradually increase the movement your arms will "fly" up to your shoulders. Slowly reduce the twisting, at the same speed as you increased it. When you stop you will feel you are still moving.

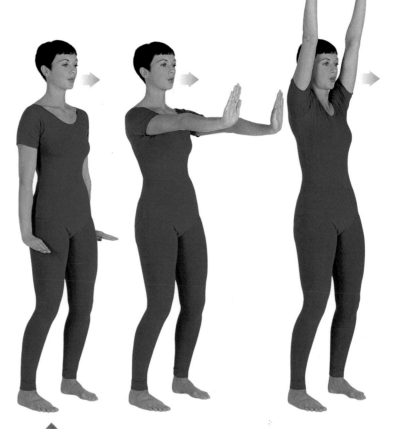

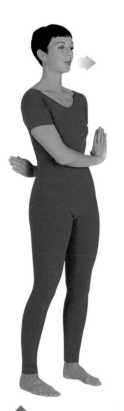

3 Exhale and pause while you move your right arm, palm upright, across your body to the left. Inhale as your left arm moves to your back. Again, imagine pushing soft clouds away from you on both sides. Exhale and repeat with your left arm in front.

Breathing impulse

There is no special impulse necessary when we "let go the air" – that is, breathe out. It is a relaxed movement made easy by the laws of gravity. Breathing in, on the other hand, activates the whole body and is an automatic impulse triggered by the brain. When the blood lacks oxygen, the breathing muscles are "ordered" to contract causing the in-breath.

4 On an out-breath push your arms down, with palms outstretched, then raise them up in front and lift them above your head in a semicircle. Keep your knees slightly bent to allow this swinging movement to take hold of your whole body.

5 With your whole body feeling ▶ comfortably stretched breathe in and move arms to shoulder height with palms upright. Breathe out, push away the clouds. Repeat steps 4 and 5 twice.

6 Inhale and keep your arms stretched before you exhale and let them come to rest at your sides. Breathe on impulse, softly rocking on your cloud. Watch the movement of your breath and note how much space is now provided for it in your breathing areas.

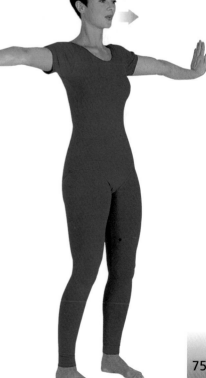

75

The Root

Duration: 20 minutes.

Aim:
To strengthen and stabilize breathing areas 1 and 2.

Mental attitude:
Ready for challenges – not to be stopped by any resistance.

Positive side-effects:
Strengthening and stretching leg muscles; mobilizing hip and knee joints; stimulating circulation.

Ultimate effect:
Feel the air flowing vigorously into legs and feet; increased fitness.

Breathing takes root in our bodies. In the five sequences of this exercise you challenge yourself to explore your breath beyond its manifestation in the breathing areas. You will become aware of the stimulation of all your body activities which takes place every time you breathe. With each in-breath the powerful flow moves from the diaphragm to the pelvis to the legs and feet and into the floor you are standing on. This conjures up the image of "taking root" and this instant contact with the floor gives you stability.

Strength and stability. . .1

1 Rest with your legs out in front of you, then put your soles on the floor. Breathe in and out and become aware of the rhythm of your breath. With every out-breath gently let your shoulders and lumbar spine sink into the floor.

Starting position –
Supine
page 28

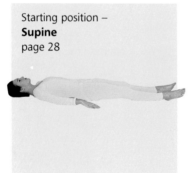

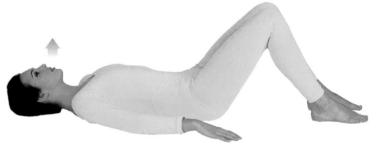

2 Breathe out and push your right leg away from your body along the floor. Use your hip to help you stretch. Breathe in and pull your leg back. Repeat using your left leg. Repeat this three times for each leg. ▼

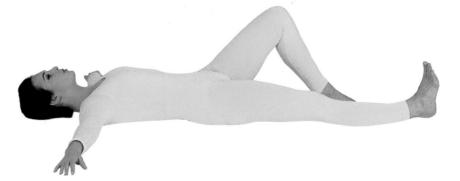

3 Breathe out again and at the end of the out-breath push your legs and heels away from you while pulling the tips of your toes toward you. You should feel the tension along the length of your legs, from heel to hip. ▼

4 Inhale and roll up your pelvis ▶ until you can feel the flow of air filling breathing area 1 – not beyond the point where your groin muscles are stretched and your thighs and trunk form one line. Breathe out and roll back, vertebra by vertebra.

5 Repeat; then breathe in and move your arms up, too, in a semicircle on the floor. Your elbows should stay in contact with the floor, otherwise the tension in your shoulders will be uncomfortable. Slowly move your arms back to shoulder level while exhaling. ▼

6 Breathe out and push your right leg away from you (as step 2); at the same time stretch your left arm up. When you feel your leg is sprouting out of you push your arm further, away from the shoulder joint. The lumbar spine is supported by your other leg but remains flexible. You are stretched diagonally. ▼

7 Breathe in, then return to the starting position while breathing out. Inhale and repeat with your left leg and right arm.

Strength and stability. . .2

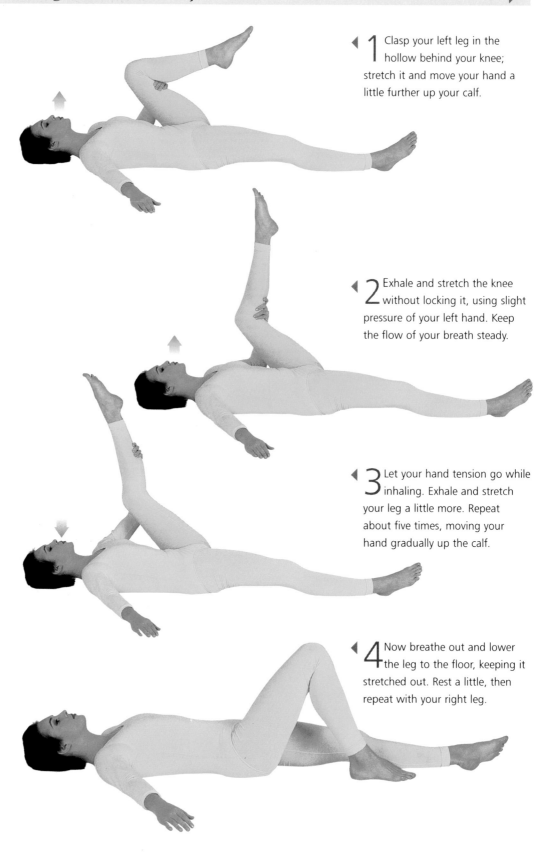

◀ 1 Clasp your left leg in the hollow behind your knee; stretch it and move your hand a little further up your calf.

◀ 2 Exhale and stretch the knee without locking it, using slight pressure of your left hand. Keep the flow of your breath steady.

◀ 3 Let your hand tension go while inhaling. Exhale and stretch your leg a little more. Repeat about five times, moving your hand gradually up the calf.

◀ 4 Now breathe out and lower the leg to the floor, keeping it stretched out. Rest a little, then repeat with your right leg.

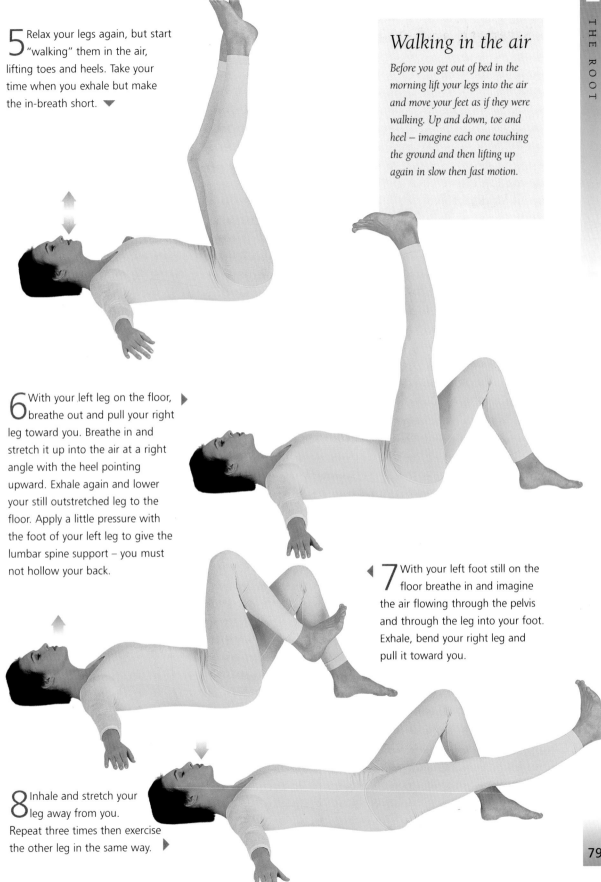

5 Relax your legs again, but start "walking" them in the air, lifting toes and heels. Take your time when you exhale but make the in-breath short. ▼

Walking in the air

Before you get out of bed in the morning lift your legs into the air and move your feet as if they were walking. Up and down, toe and heel – imagine each one touching the ground and then lifting up again in slow then fast motion.

6 With your left leg on the floor, ▶ breathe out and pull your right leg toward you. Breathe in and stretch it up into the air at a right angle with the heel pointing upward. Exhale again and lower your still outstretched leg to the floor. Apply a little pressure with the foot of your left leg to give the lumbar spine support – you must not hollow your back.

7 With your left foot still on the floor breathe in and imagine the air flowing through the pelvis and through the leg into your foot. Exhale, bend your right leg and pull it toward you.

8 Inhale and stretch your leg away from you. Repeat three times then exercise the other leg in the same way. ▶

Strength and stability. . . 3

1 Clasp the fronts of your knees with your hands. Breathe out and pull them toward your chest. Let go of your knees, breathe in and stretch out your legs. ▶

2 Place your hands across the hollow at the back of your knees, then exhale and pull your outstretched legs toward you.

3 Release the tension on your legs while inhaling then pull them down again, drawing them a little closer to your chest each time. Repeat this as long as you want, not forcing the movement. ▶

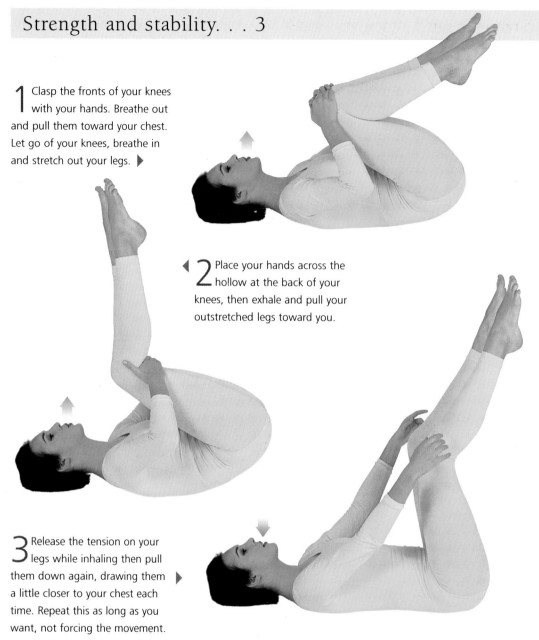

4 Keep your legs stretched and breathe in. Breathe out and swiftly roll yourself up into a sitting position – you will come to rest on your bent legs.

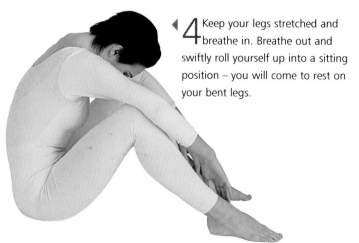

Relax into it

Make sure your back is soft and your shoulders are relaxed. It helps if you move your elbows to the sides whenever you pull your legs toward you, whether they are bent or stretched. This will prevent your shoulders from moving upward. Keep your head aligned with your body.

Strength and stability. . . 4

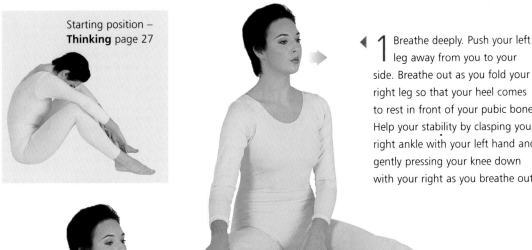

Starting position –
Thinking page 27

1 Breathe deeply. Push your left leg away from you to your side. Breathe out as you fold your right leg so that your heel comes to rest in front of your pubic bone. Help your stability by clasping your right ankle with your left hand and gently pressing your knee down with your right as you breathe out.

2 Inhale and turn your leg so the calf comes to rest alongside the right thigh. Exhale and gently press your knee down with your left hand and your ankle with your right hand. Your trunk should be erect. Repeat up to five times this stretches your thigh muscles and gives mobility to your hip joint. It allows free passage of air into breathing areas 1 and 2 and the pelvis. Repeat with your other leg.

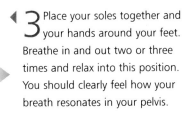

3 Place your soles together and your hands around your feet. Breathe in and out two or three times and relax into this position. You should clearly feel how your breath resonates in your pelvis.

4 When you breathe out shift your weight to the pelvis. Bend forward, clasp your feet with your hands, breathe out and slowly push your feet away. Always stretch the legs when you exhale.

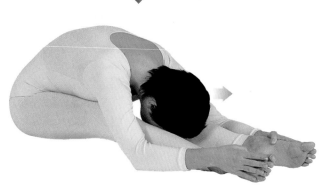

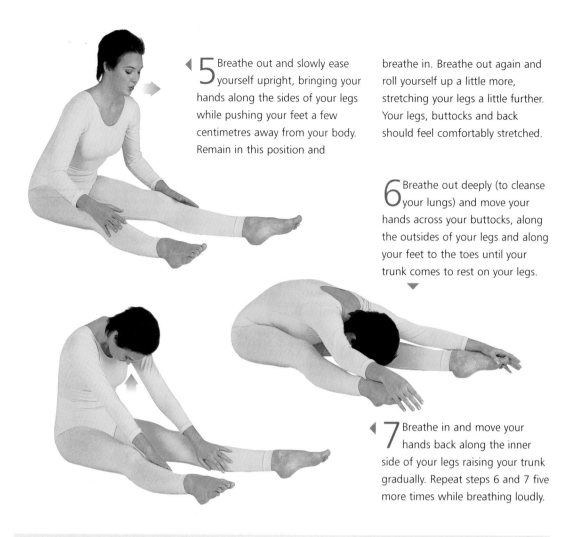

◄ 5 Breathe out and slowly ease yourself upright, bringing your hands along the sides of your legs while pushing your feet a few centimetres away from your body. Remain in this position and breathe in. Breathe out again and roll yourself up a little more, stretching your legs a little further. Your legs, buttocks and back should feel comfortably stretched.

6 Breathe out deeply (to cleanse your lungs) and move your hands across your buttocks, along the outsides of your legs and along your feet to the toes until your trunk comes to rest on your legs. ▼

◄ 7 Breathe in and move your hands back along the inner side of your legs raising your trunk gradually. Repeat steps 6 and 7 five more times while breathing loudly.

Strength and stability. . .5 ▶

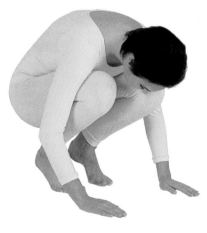

1 Crouch with your soles firmly on the floor. Balance on your toes, bend your trunk forward and place your hands in front of you. Breathe out several times.

2 Place soles flat, breathe in. Each time you exhale raise ▶ your pelvis by stretching your legs a little at a time. Pause and breathe in between stretches. When the knees are fully stretched. the top half of your body will be almost parallel with the bottom half, your head lies on your knees. The closer your hands are to your feet the stronger the tension in the leg muscles at the back.

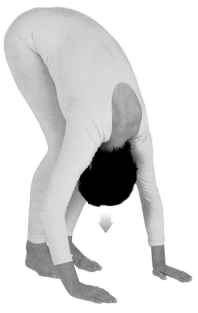

3 Bend your knees a little and let your trunk hang loosely. Breathe in and out two to three times before you roll yourself up, vertebra by vertebra, to a standing position with arms hanging loosely. ▼

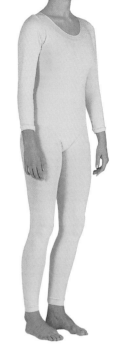

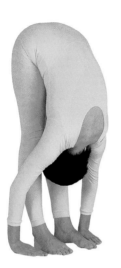

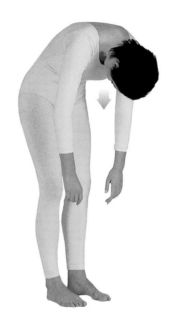

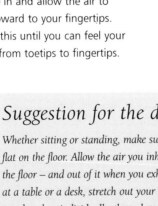

4 Breathe in and stretch your arms upward, bring them back down in opposite directions while breathing out. Your arms are describing a circle – this may take practice to achieve. Get your strength from the floor when you breathe in and allow the air to flow upward to your fingertips. Repeat this until you can feel your breath from toetips to fingertips.

5 Finish by standing still, becoming aware once again of having taken root. Breathe out and relax. ▶

Suggestion for the day

Whether sitting or standing, make sure your soles rest flat on the floor. Allow the air you inhale to flow into the floor – and out of it when you exhale. When sitting at a table or a desk, stretch out your legs frequently, together then individually, then place feet flat again.

The Flower

Duration: 20 minutes.

Aim:
Expanding breathing areas 2, 3 and 4 by stretching (especially breathing areas 2 and 4).

Mental attitude:
Be ready to open up like a flower, slowly and gradually.

Positive side-effects:
Balancing the spine; correcting the posture by opening up the ribcage and stretching the back to achieve a correct posture; taking the strain off the heart.

Ultimate effect:
A controlled and open chest area. The breath has expanded, gained in volume and space.

Flowers open up when it is warm and light, when the roots can draw strength from the soil. For the four sequences in this exercise, create a light, warm atmosphere around yourself. A sense of stability is needed and the aim is to give your lungs space to breathe so they work at full capacity. You activate them, expand them inside and out so air reaches muscles and tissue unhindered.

Always make sure your movements are smooth. Increase the pace of them gradually – a flower grows slowly and blossoms when nurtured and encouraged.

Extend and stretch. . .1 ▶

1 When you have found a comfortable position on your back, spread out your arms, bend your knees and place your feet firmly on the floor. ▼

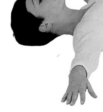

Starting position

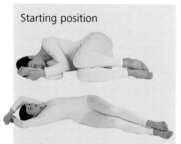

Lie down on the floor as if you were about to go to sleep, slightly curled up. Breathe in and out a few times. Breathe out strongly and try to shift the whole of your body weight to the floor. Once you feel really comfortable and are in contact with your breathing, start waking up, stretching your arms and legs in all directions. Yawn, roll from one side to the other.

2 Become aware of the rhythm of your breath. With each out-breath lightly swing your knees from side to side. Apply a little pressure with the foot that stays on the floor for stability. Give in to the impulse to breathe in. ▼

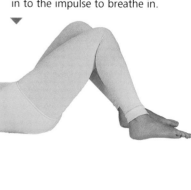

3 Lower your legs just a little, then increase the swinging movement gradually on breathing out. Give in a little to the tension you feel to stretch breathing area 2 slightly. Swing your legs in this way until you can clearly feel your breath in breathing areas 1 and 2. Your shoulders and arms should be relaxed and resting on the floor. Place both feet flat and breathe deeply. Now turn your attention to breathing areas 3 and 4.

4 Breathe in and push each arm in turn further out, making sure the movement is in tune with the rhythm of your breath. You will notice that your shoulder blades also move sideward. Keep on stretching and slowly, centimetre by centimetre, move your arms upward without lifting them – your elbows must not lose contact with the floor.

5 The higher you move your arms with each in-breath the more clearly you will feel your ribs in breathing areas 3 and 4 (in the whole of your ribcage) opening up and closing like a fan. Stop before it becomes uncomfortable.

6 Inhale and stretch both your arms to your fingertips. Remain in this position for a moment, then exhale, bringing your arms back to shoulder level.

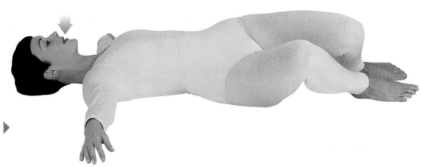

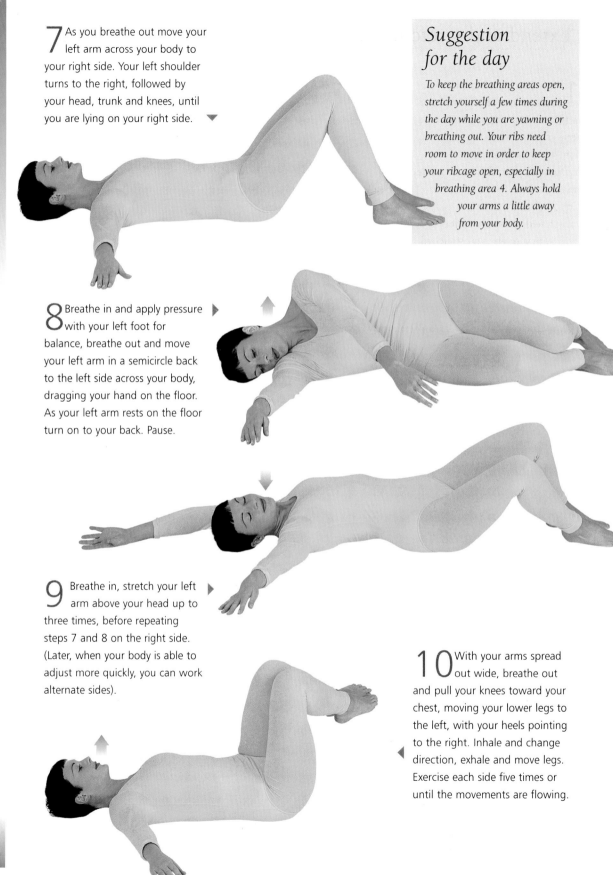

7 As you breathe out move your left arm across your body to your right side. Your left shoulder turns to the right, followed by your head, trunk and knees, until you are lying on your right side. ▼

Suggestion for the day

To keep the breathing areas open, stretch yourself a few times during the day while you are yawning or breathing out. Your ribs need room to move in order to keep your ribcage open, especially in breathing area 4. Always hold your arms a little away from your body.

8 Breathe in and apply pressure with your left foot for balance, breathe out and move your left arm in a semicircle back to the left side across your body, dragging your hand on the floor. As your left arm rests on the floor turn on to your back. Pause.

9 Breathe in, stretch your left arm above your head up to three times, before repeating steps 7 and 8 on the right side. (Later, when your body is able to adjust more quickly, you can work alternate sides).

10 With your arms spread out wide, breathe out and pull your knees toward your chest, moving your lower legs to the left, with your heels pointing to the right. Inhale and change direction, exhale and move legs. Exercise each side five times or until the movements are flowing.

Extend and stretch. . .2

1 Raise your right leg, place your left foot on the knee and rest. Breathe in and out three times, then gently stretch your right leg along the floor. Breathe out and use your left foor to guide your right knee to the left. Your hip follows the movement, but your shoulders remain on the floor, with your arms outstretched.

Note: If you suffer from irregularities in the lumbar spine or you find this exercise painful try circling your pulled-up knees when resting.

2 Exhale and try to press your right knee as close to the floor as possible. Inhale and pull your left knee toward your chest then exhale, raise your right leg again and briskly repeat steps 1 and 2.

3 Now turn your body to the right, with your left arm following and describing a semicircle until it comes to rest outstretched on your other arm. Your left leg lies on the floor, both knees are bent. Breathe freely.

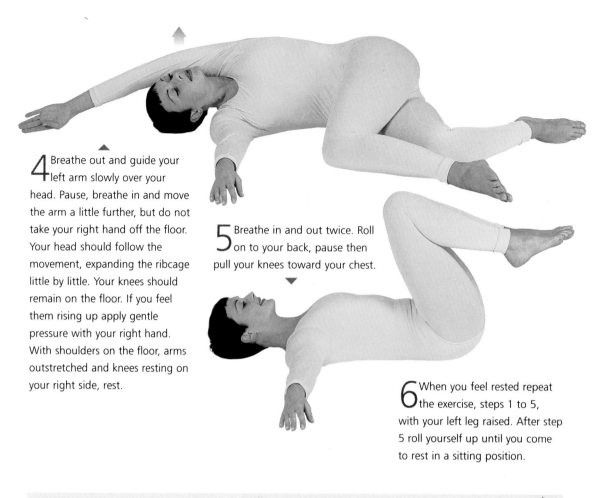

4 Breathe out and guide your left arm slowly over your head. Pause, breathe in and move the arm a little further, but do not take your right hand off the floor. Your head should follow the movement, expanding the ribcage little by little. Your knees should remain on the floor. If you feel them rising up apply gentle pressure with your right hand. With shoulders on the floor, arms outstretched and knees resting on your right side, rest.

5 Breathe in and out twice. Roll on to your back, pause then pull your knees toward your chest.

6 When you feel rested repeat the exercise, steps 1 to 5, with your left leg raised. After step 5 roll yourself up until you come to rest in a sitting position.

Extend and stretch. . .3

Starting position –
Thinking
page 27

Make sure breathing areas 3 and 4 remain open.

1 Straddle your legs in front of you. Breathing out, move your left arm in a semicircle toward your right foot, then swing it to your left and roll yourself upright keeping your buttocks firmly on the floor. Your right hand provides support. ▼

Take your time

Many flowers – like the evening primrose – can take a long time for the petals to open so take your time. Try and expand the movement a little each day. If you feel a lot of tension in breathing area 4 (above the armpit), take a few breaths and rest a moment. When you breathe out let go a little in order to stimulate the muscles to stretch themselves.

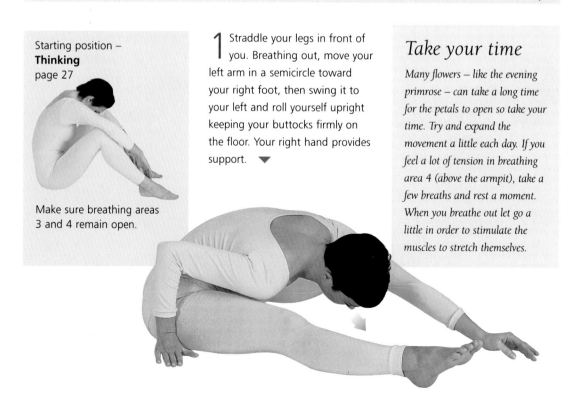

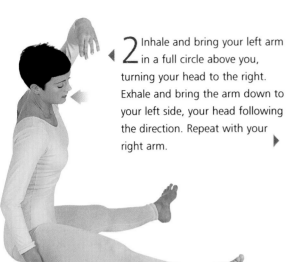

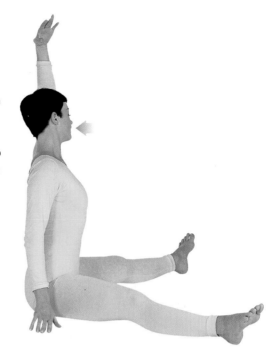

2 Inhale and bring your left arm in a full circle above you, turning your head to the right. Exhale and bring the arm down to your left side, your head following the direction. Repeat with your right arm.

3 Breathe out and swing both arms forward, clasping hands. Breathe in, pull yourself upright and open up the arms above your head. Repeat several times, but make sure the pelvis remains on the floor. Breathe out, bring arms down in a semicircle to the side.

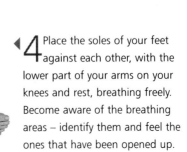

4 Place the soles of your feet against each other, with the lower part of your arms on your knees and rest, breathing freely. Become aware of the breathing areas – identify them and feel the ones that have been opened up.

Extend and stretch. . .4

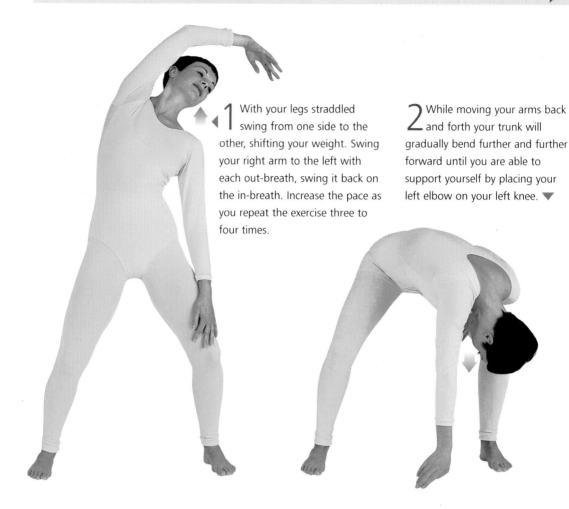

1 With your legs straddled swing from one side to the other, shifting your weight. Swing your right arm to the left with each out-breath, swing it back on the in-breath. Increase the pace as you repeat the exercise three to four times.

2 While moving your arms back and forth your trunk will gradually bend further and further forward until you are able to support yourself by placing your left elbow on your left knee. ▼

Breathing states

When you breathe out, your mind influences your physical self with the aim of bringing an overall feeling of relaxation. Phrases used to describe this state are: to let go, to lay down, to give way, to relax, to become weak, to pour out, to empty, to give, to rest. The longer and slower the out-breath, the more relaxed your body will be.

4 Swing both your arms down to the floor on an out-breath (your knees will bend), then swing them high above your head on an in-breath (your knees will stretch).

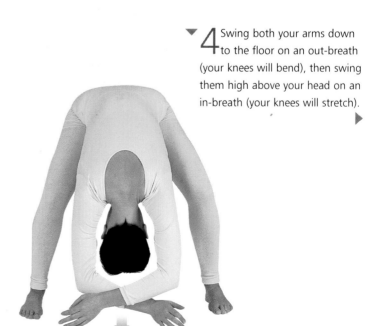

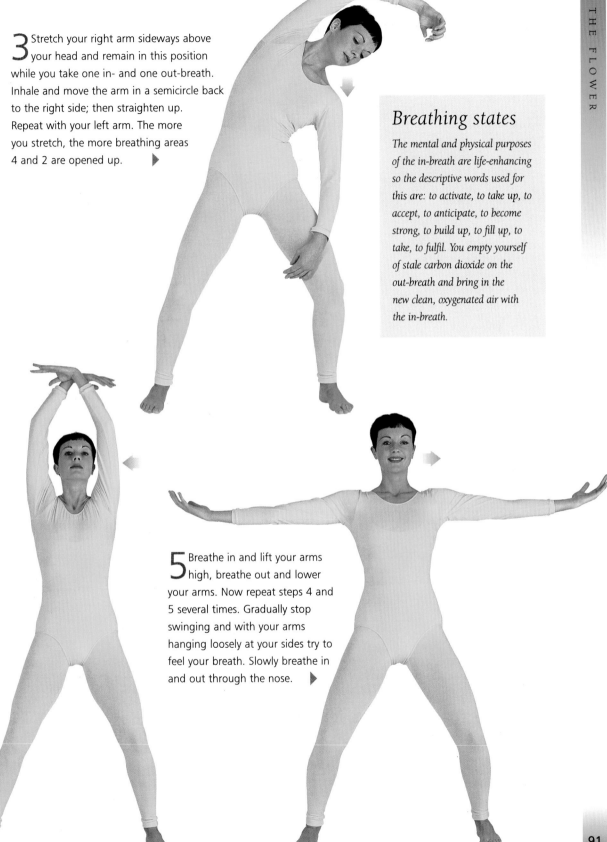

3 Stretch your right arm sideways above your head and remain in this position while you take one in- and one out-breath. Inhale and move the arm in a semicircle back to the right side; then straighten up. Repeat with your left arm. The more you stretch, the more breathing areas 4 and 2 are opened up. ▶

Breathing states

The mental and physical purposes of the in-breath are life-enhancing so the descriptive words used for this are: to activate, to take up, to accept, to anticipate, to become strong, to build up, to fill up, to take, to fulfil. You empty yourself of stale carbon dioxide on the out-breath and bring in the new clean, oxygenated air with the in-breath.

5 Breathe in and lift your arms high, breathe out and lower your arms. Now repeat steps 4 and 5 several times. Gradually stop swinging and with your arms hanging loosely at your sides try to feel your breath. Slowly breathe in and out through the nose. ▶

The Ball

Duration: 10 minutes.

Aim:
To become aware of the
breathing reflex and learn to
give in to it.

Mental attitude:
Become a ball; exercise briskly,
at different speeds.

Positive side-effects:
Fitness training for the whole
body; strengthening the
abdomen, lower back,
buttocks and legs.

Ultimate effect:
Strengthening, vitalizing;
increased alertness.

This exercise has five sequences which deal with the reflex, impulsive breathing that follows after you have been exercising. The effect it has on the body can be illustrated by the way the elastic walls of a ball contract and quickly expand in play. The movement of the breath reflects this tension which is felt in the way the diaphragm reacts.

It is important throughout the exercise that you do not consciously inhale but allow it to occur naturally in response to the body's need for air. This keeps the muscular diaphragm exercised, so it contracts well when you breathe out and relaxes when you breathe in, allowing the lungs to push out the stale air and fill up again with the new. You discover the instinctive breathing reflex in which the whole body – relaxed, springy and elastic – must be involved, not just the nose, throat, lungs and chest.

Before you start

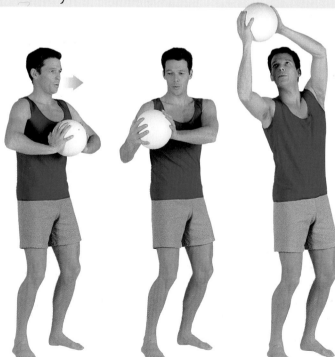

Hold a plastic beach ball or blown-up balloon between your hands. Breathe out and slightly squeeze the ball, bending your knees as you do so. When the walls of the ball expand again you should feel the impulse to breathe in.

Try this several times applying different pressure but don't force it. Feel the tension, and act on it. Exhale through the mouth making these sounds: "sh", "s", "f". This slows down the flow of air and you will feel tension in the diaphragm.

Feel your breathing

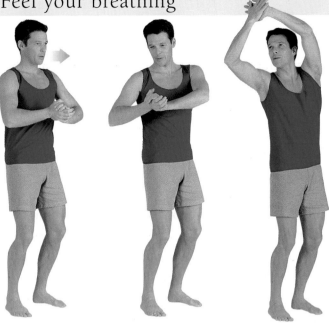

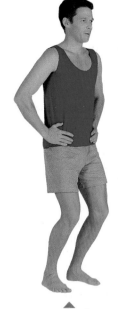

1 Press your hands against each other, feel the slight resistance. Breathe out and press hands, release the pressure with the in-breath. This movement is reflected in the knees, which you bend but never completely stretch again. Repeat the actions with the arms in different positions until you have mastered the breathing rhythm.

2 Place your palms on your hips. With each out-breath press your hands against your pelvis. Release the pressure when you feel the impulse to breathe in. Do this three times.

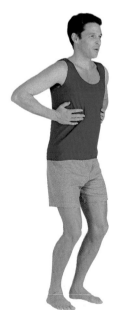

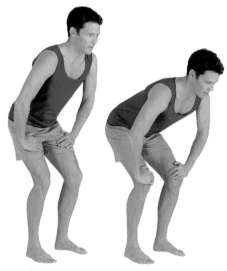

5 As in step 4, move your hands down the back of your lower legs to your ankles. Clasp them from the back, breathe out and pull your trunk between your knees. Breathe on impulse. ▼

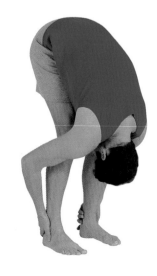

3 Move on to breathing area 3, lightly pressing the ribcage and diaphragm with each out-breath. This is the base of your breathing reflex.

4 Now feel breathing areas 2 and 1. Bend your knees, press your hands along your thighs, step by step to your knees. Rest there, breathing in and out a few times. Bend your knees on an out-breath, slightly stretch them on inhaling.

Breathe and bounce. . .1

Suggestion for the day

Try to remember not to slouch – in every respect! Bounce up and down whenever you can. If this is not possible, take a few breaths, sniffing the air to feel your breathing impulses.

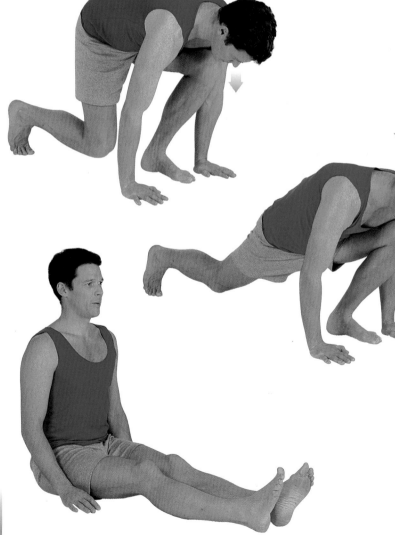

1 Place your hands flat on the floor in front of you and crouch down. Breathe out and bounce up and down on springy joints, just like a ball, keeping your hands on the floor. When the reflex impulse to breathe in occurs listen to your breath – it should be a soft sound, not harsh.

2 Keeping your bouncing momentum, move your right leg backward along the floor little by little on a long out-breath. After about five bounces your leg will be fully extended. Keep your hands on the floor, inhale on demand. Breathing out, pull the leg back in again – step by step – and bounce a little every time you move it.

3 Repeat with your left leg. Remain crouched. With your hands behind your knees for support, bounce – down on the out-breath, up on the in-breath. Increase the pace as long as you feel comfortable.

4 Sit down to rest; stretch your legs out in front and pretend you are walking. Breathe freely.

Breathe and bounce. . .2

1 Breathe deeply then bend your left knee, clasp it with your left hand and "bounce" it toward your body five times each time you exhale. Imagine you are squeezing a balloon placed between your knee and your chest. You can even use a balloon if you like. Ensure your trunk is upright. Note how your whole spine is stretched.

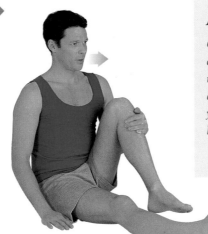

Are you ready?

Only attempt the sequence shown on this page if your stomach muscles are well-exercised – and only if you have managed to feel your breath clearly in both breathing areas 1 and 2.

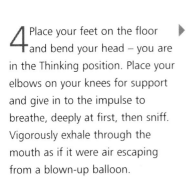

2 Pulling both your knees toward your body, repeat the exercise with both knees, "bouncing" your feet along the floor as you breathe out.

3 Clasp the back of your thighs ▶ with your hands and pull your knees toward your chest. Your feet will lift off the floor; your weight is on your sitting bones and sacrum. Find the right balance and make sure you can feel your breath.

4 Place your feet on the floor ▶ and bend your head – you are in the Thinking position. Place your elbows on your knees for support and give in to the impulse to breathe, deeply at first, then sniff. Vigorously exhale through the mouth as if it were air escaping from a blown-up balloon.

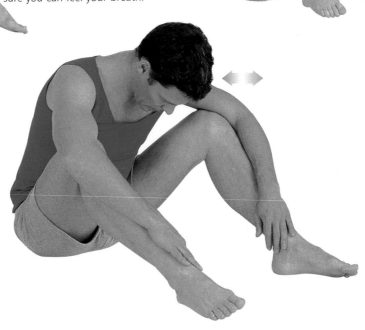

Tense and stretch

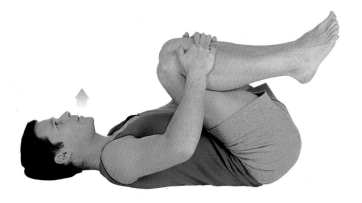

1 Lie on your back and breathe ▶
deeply. Breathe out, clasp your
bent knees and pull them to your
chest, feeling the elastic tension
everywhere but especially in the
walls of the diaphragm – as if you
were squeezing the ball hard.
When you give in to the impulse to
inhale, relax your arms. Breathing
out, pull each knee alternately to
your chest several times. ▶

A good grasp

*If you cannot reach your heels at
first (see step 6 opposite), try
clasping the ankles or the calves.
The eventual aim is to be able to
grasp your heels.*

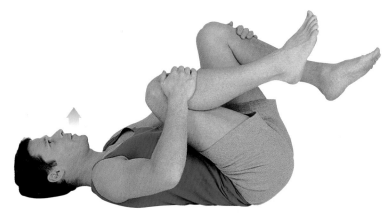

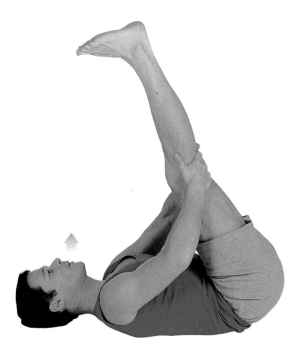

◀ 2 Stretch your legs into the air,
clasping them at the back of
the knees. Breathing out, pull the
right leg, then the left leg, then
both legs together toward you.
Repeat this quickly three times –
first, with stretched legs, then with
bent knees. Your back should feel
soft before you pull the bent knees
toward you while exhaling. Breathe
in, stretch your legs and, with the
help of your hands, pull the
stretched-out legs toward you.

3 Repeat step 2 a few times until you feel mobile. With each out-breath try and pull the legs further and further back, toes behind your head, until your thighs are parallel to the floor. The pelvis is lifted off the floor.

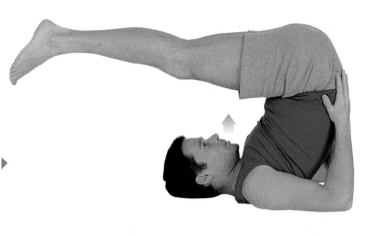

4 Place your hands at the back between your pelvis and ribcage with upper arms on the floor for support. Keep your legs outstretched and bounce them downward a few times – your breathing keeps pace. ▶

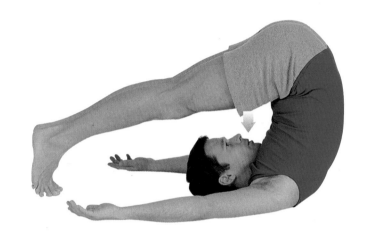

5 Pause and press your toes to the floor with your arms stretched above your head (or by your side). Wait for the impulse to breathe, then on an out-breath bring your legs back to the Supine position. Now roll yourself upward into a sitting position with your legs wide apart. ▶

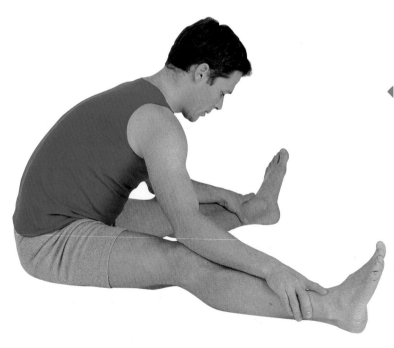

◀ 6 Clasp your legs at the lowest possible point (preferably the heels) and pull your abdomen down with every out-breath, then pull it to the right, to the left and down again. Remain sitting, legs outstretched, and wait for the impulse to breathe. On an out-breath, sit upright with your hands on your thighs. Relax and breathe freely.

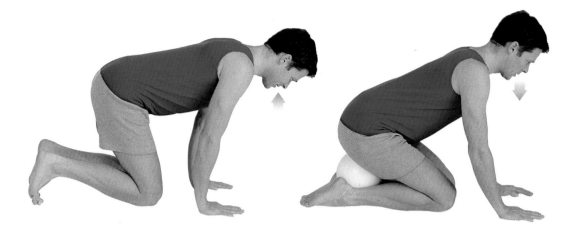

Tense and bounce

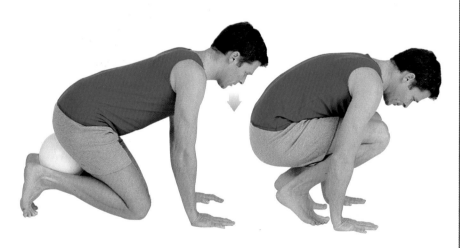

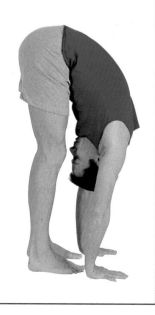

1 Get on to all fours and breathe freely. Imagine there is a ball balanced on your heels. When you breathe out you are sitting back on this ball – but when you breathe in on impulse it bounces you back on to all fours.

2 Now do the exercise with a beach ball in place. Bounce your buttocks on to your heels, bounce up a little, then bounce back down on to the right heel, then the left, then both. Continue like this until the breathing reflex is so natural that you feel you never want to stop.

3 Bounce up and down again a few times, until your toes are pointing downward (and the ball is released). Now get back into a crouching position with your feet under you and hands on the floor.

4 Breathe deeply and sniff. This breathing reflex not only loosens and tones the diaphragm but also makes you more alert and gives you more energy.

Hands down

The aim of step 5 (right) is to keep your hands flat on the floor and knees stretched between bounces, but you might not be able to do this the first time you try. If you practise regularly you will achieve this position easily. Your body should stay soft and you should stretch as far as you can without it becoming painful or causing strain.

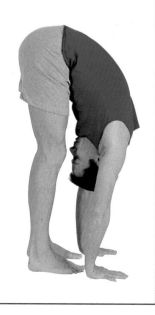

5 Keeping your palms and feet on the floor, bounce yourself upward – as if you were a ball being bounced – in three to five movements on each out-breath. Try to straighten the knees a little more on each movement.

6 Breathe out and begin to roll up your trunk, vertebra by vertebra. Take your time. Breathe on impulse if you like between each section of the rolling. ▼

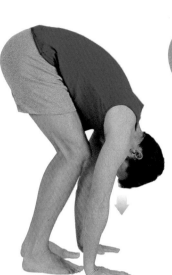 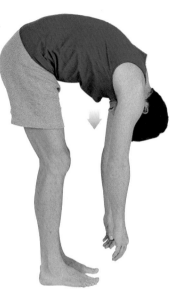 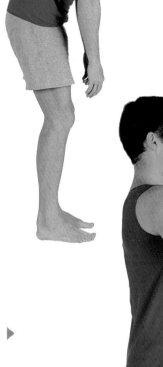

7 With a beach ball or balloon in your hands, breathe out and squeeze. Breathe in and let go of the pressure on the ball while gently stretching your trunk by pushing your arms away from your body and above your head. Go at your own pace; this exercise is very stimulating and you will certainly feel the movement in the the ligaments of the diaphragm.

8 Slightly bend your knees and press on the ball. Exhale and bounce up and down on your toes; you should hear your breath. Pause for breath and slow down. Sniff and continue bouncing on your toes, keeping upright. Stretch your spine, from the sacrum to the top of your head, and focus on it.

9 Drop your heels, stop sniffing and breathe normally. Feel the movement of your breath in your body and your impulse to breathe. Enjoy the tingling feeling in your leg and arm muscles which indicates increased energy.

The Wave

Duration:
10 minutes maximum.

Aim:
To expand and deepen full effective breathing in its various intensive stages.

Positive side-effects:
Stimulation of the blood circulation; counter-balancing and stabilizing the spine and the muscles to achieve a correct posture.

Ultimate effect:
A wave of breath recognized in all breathing areas.

With each breath you take your body is "rinsed" by a wave of oxygen. When you exhale, the breath carries away stale air lacking in oxygen. It also transmits your energy to the outside world. This wave is constant as you will find in these three sequences. Which parts of the body it reaches depends on the willingness and readiness of mind and body to allow the air to flow freely. The depth of your breathing also depends on your ability to tune in to your inner being.

In the previous nine exercises you have learned to become aware of yourself and your breath. If the wave ripples gently, the breathing will be shallow. If the breath comes in big waves and the breathing areas are opened up, you receive energy. All you have to do now is to allow the wave of breath to flow in and stop it when necessary.

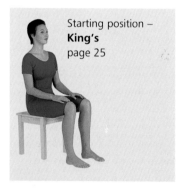

Starting position –
King's
page 25

Rhythm and rolling ▶

1 Let your arms hang at your sides and slightly stretch your neck. Start rolling your spine from top to bottom, vertebra by vertebra, rolling with every out-breath. Take your time and stop whenever you need to breathe in.

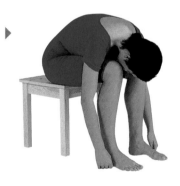

Making waves

Physiologically the wave of oxygen is caused by the interplay of muscles in the chest and ribcage which makes the thoracic cavity greater or smaller and makes the lungs fill or empty themselves. The bigger the wave the more you will feel the effect on your body.

2 Breathe out and slowly lower your head; you will feel your neck slightly stretching. Roll from the thoracic spine to the base of the diaphragm. When you reach the lumbar spine your trunk will be bent deep down, with your arms loose at your sides. When you roll the lower spine your trunk will rest on your thighs.

3 Remain in this position and breathe in and out two to three times. When you breathe out shift the weight of your trunk to your thighs. When you pause the inner tension will be released. Take two to three breaths on impulse.

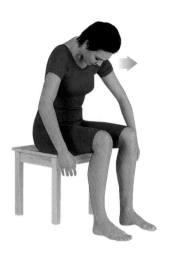

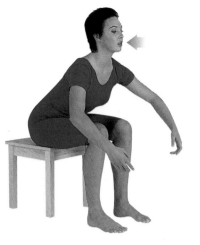

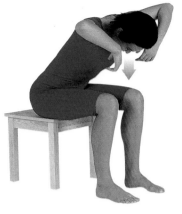

4 Become aware of the wave of your breath before you guide it to the movement you are performing. At first it is small, only to be felt in the lower back. Then it spreads from breathing area 1 through the whole trunk beyond the breathing areas to the top of your cervical spine and your head.

5 With each in-breath roll yourself up a little. Breathe out and do not move but let go a little by allowing the movement to accompany the outgoing breath.

6 Use your arms to help the air flow. Breathe in and guide the inside of your hand (thumb and forefinger) along the side of your body and beyond until the arms are stretched above your head. When you have finished breathing in your arms are stretched, your head moved back a little. Breathe out and lower your arms in a semicircle to your side, keeping them slightly arched.

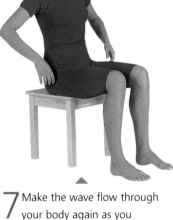

7 Make the wave flow through your body again as you breathe in and out once. With your mind, follow the wave from breathing area 1 to breathing area 3 and still further on, into your head. Exhale the air slowly through pursed lips.

8 Inhale and straighten up. Arms stretched, bend forward while exhaling until your trunk rests on your thighs then breathe out the rest of the air. Arch your arms and move them to the front. Breathe in and straighten up, supported by a littl foot pressure. Repeat two to three times.

9 Now bend forward a little less each time you breathe out. When you breathe in stretch yourself and feel comfortable doing it. Bend your trunk less and less until you are almost still. Inhale and remain for a moment with outstretched arms and your trunk comfortably stretched.

10 Slowly guide the out-breath and lower your arms at the same time in a wide curve. When all air is exhaled your arms should rest at your sides, not touching the body. Remain in this position and breathe deeply.

Extend your breathing

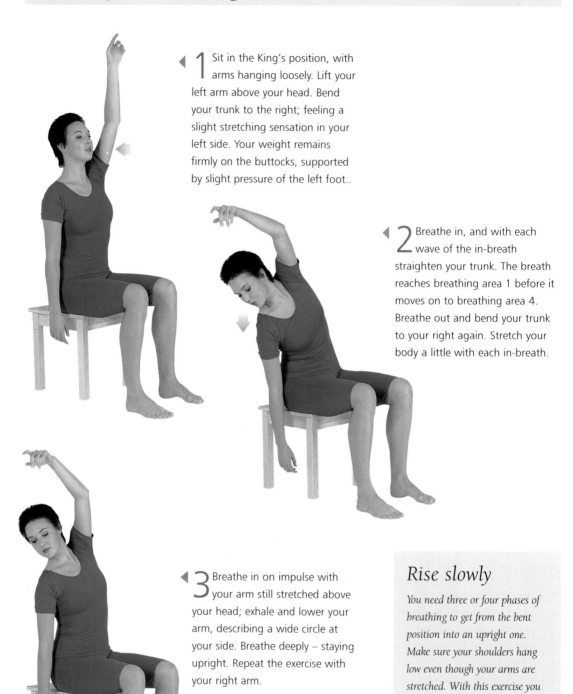

1 Sit in the King's position, with arms hanging loosely. Lift your left arm above your head. Bend your trunk to the right; feeling a slight stretching sensation in your left side. Your weight remains firmly on the buttocks, supported by slight pressure of the left foot..

2 Breathe in, and with each wave of the in-breath straighten your trunk. The breath reaches breathing area 1 before it moves on to breathing area 4. Breathe out and bend your trunk to your right again. Stretch your body a little with each in-breath.

3 Breathe in on impulse with your arm still stretched above your head; exhale and lower your arm, describing a wide circle at your side. Breathe deeply – staying upright. Repeat the exercise with your right arm.

Rise slowly

You need three or four phases of breathing to get from the bent position into an upright one. Make sure your shoulders hang low even though your arms are stretched. With this exercise you stabilize your posture when breathing out. Keep your trunk upright when exhaling and keep the breathing areas open.

4 Let the wave from the side ▶
and the one from the front
come together. Breathe out and
bend forward, breathe in and
quickly straighten up. The arms
accompany this movement.
Immediately lower your right arm
but leave your left arm loosely
stretched above your head.

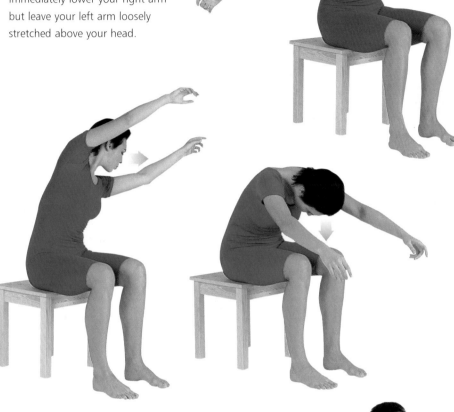

5 Exhale and bend to the left,
both arms following the
movement. Inhale and straighten
up again. Change direction of the

arms. Bend forward with arms out
in front, breathe in and straighten
up. Repeat steps 4 and 5 (now
with arms to the right).

6 Return to the King's position ▶
and breathe on impulse. You
should feel all the breathing areas
flooded with the wave of breath. If
you cannot feel breathing area 4
well, repeat this sequence before
you move on.

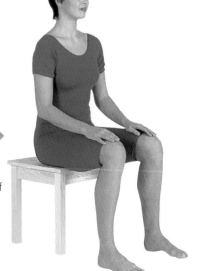

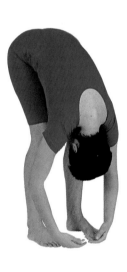

Rolling out tension

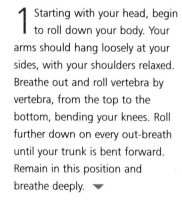

1 Starting with your head, begin to roll down your body. Your arms should hang loosely at your sides, with your shoulders relaxed. Breathe out and roll vertebra by vertebra, from the top to the bottom, bending your knees. Roll further down on every out-breath until your trunk is bent forward. Remain in this position and breathe deeply. ▼

2 Inhale and start rolling yourself upward from the sacrum. Keep your knees flexed. Exhale and stretch the trunk forward – from the buttocks to the head – at the same time stretch your arms forward on either side of your head. When you have finished exhaling stretch your hands forward. Imagine air flowing out. ▼

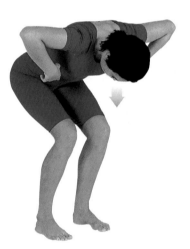

Before you start

Stand upright with your legs hip-width apart, soles flat on the floor. Breathe out and shift the weight of your body to the floor. When you next breathe in follow the wave of your breath from the bottom to the top. Breathe in and out like this three times; each breath will straighten you up. Make yourself stretch even more by stretching your spine a little every time you inhale. You should feel your breath quite clearly in the abdominal area (breathing areas 1 and 2). When you feel comfortably stretched – from your soles to the top of your head – you are ready for the sequence shown on these pages.

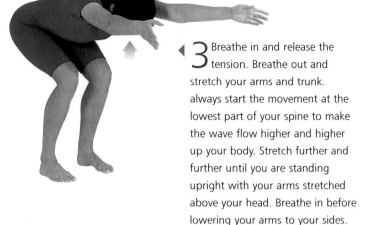

3 Breathe in and release the tension. Breathe out and stretch your arms and trunk. always start the movement at the lowest part of your spine to make the wave flow higher and higher up your body. Stretch further and further until you are standing upright with your arms stretched above your head. Breathe in before lowering your arms to your sides.

4 Breathe on impulse while standing upright. Every time you breathe in feel the wave of your breath and the extent to which your body is stretched. Increase this feeling by stretching even further, from the sacrum to the top of your head. Note that your breath must be distributed between all the breathing areas.

5 Allow the wave of breath and movement to flow briskly through your body. Enjoy the interplay of moving and being moved, of breathing in and out, of being active and letting go. Breathe out and roll your trunk forward. Give yourself a little bounce by bending your knees and pushing them forward. Then breathe in and roll yourself up, from the sacrum through to the cervical spine. The arms follow the movement; when you have finished inhaling they are stretched above your head.

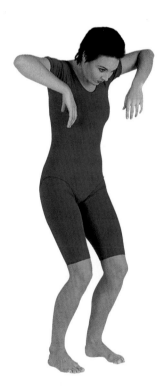

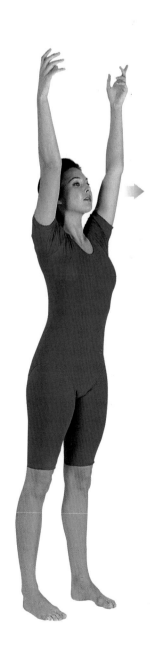

6 Exhale and bring your arms to your sides describing a semicircle; then briskly roll your trunk down, vertebra by vertebra. When the wave of the in-breath and the wave of the movement have carried you to the top remain there for a moment (arms still stretched above your head), ready to breathe in on impulse.

7 Standing upright, arms above your head, look at your posture. Allow yourself to be stretched by the wave of breath another two to three times; stretch even further when exhaling. Breathe deeply and keep the upright posture while letting go on the inside. Breathe out slowly, guiding the out-breath while lowering your arms to your sides.

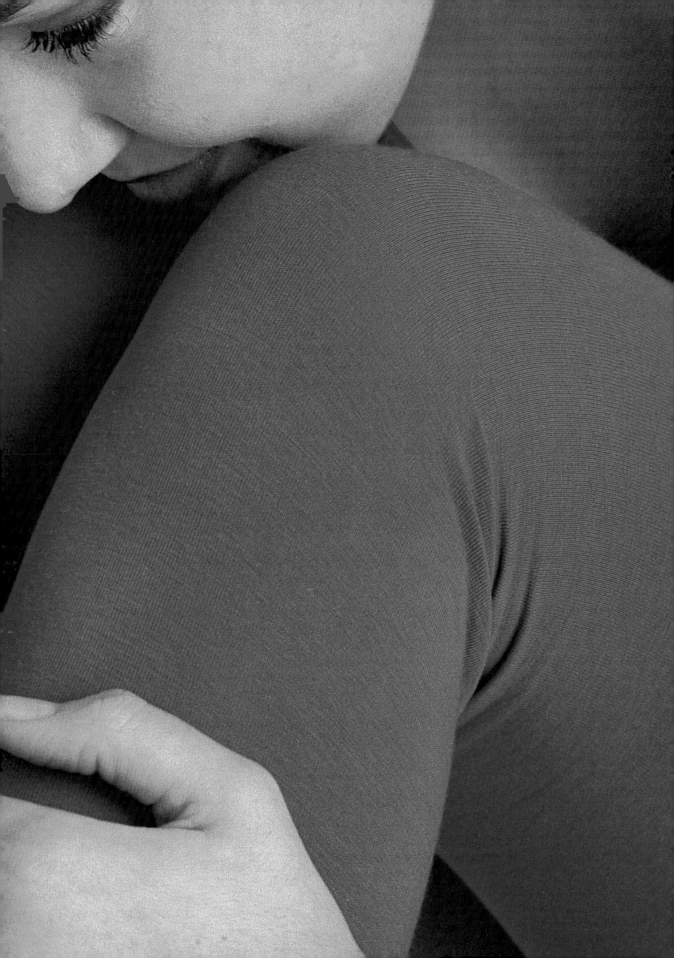

PART 3

Breathing Through the Day

Once you become conscious of the way your breathing can change its pace according to the situation you are in, you realize how much it affects the way you feel and act. Your awareness is the first step to discovering the power of breathing. By guiding and using your breath you can overcome stresses and feel a positive lift in your approach to life.

Everyday well-being

Everything you have learned from the pages in this book has just one aim – to improve your breathing to such an extent that its influence makes you feel good every minute of the day.

Even if you haven't yet had a chance to try out the breathing awareness exercises and started to appreciate the physical rewards of the training programme in Part 2, this section gives you some idea of the energy your breath can inspire and of how it can be of use in all sorts of situations.

Tiredness, irritability and lack of concentration are the most common problems people face in daily life. You have two ways of dealing with them: the first is physical, a mechanical activity; the second is mental – in which you get in touch with your breathing.

Use your breathing

You learn a lot about yourself and your feelings when you can identify the way you breathe – recognize whether it is deep, shallow, calm or agitated. With your mental powers, you can make it change.

To tackle a problem mentally you need to concentrate hard and to have a basic knowledge of the way your breath moves in your body (see pp. 14-17). In the following pages you will find tips and tricks to make you feel better, with boxes labelled "body check" and "mind check", but you may not find

these significant until you have completed some of the exercises and have felt their effects.

The activities suggested in this part can be done even with minimum understanding of the powerful role of breathing (which will come with practice). Most important is to do something for yourself each morning.

The change from sleeping to waking is enormous and if you don't pay attention to it, your body and mind suffer a shock which can lead to nervous tension. Right from the start of the day, your breathing might be hectic and irregular. It's

much better to start the day at peace with yourself and with a positive feeling of well-being.

Waking up

The way to make a difference to starting your day is to take your time from the second you open your eyes in bed. Waking up starts where you are at that moment, not after your second cup of coffee or tea. In fact, the time between waking up and sitting down to breakfast will have an influence on you and how you feel for the rest of the day. Do yourself a favour and put the alarm on 10 minutes earlier than usual and use that time to get in touch with your breath, to stimulate your circulation and get ready for the day. You will feel the benefits for hours.

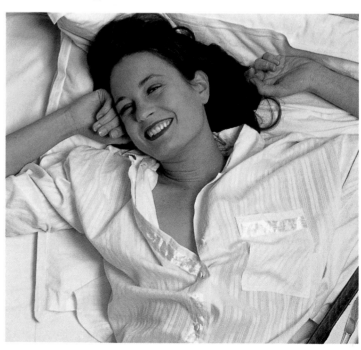

Say good morning to your system

Unless it is to answer the sound of a baby's cry, the telephone or the postman knocking at the door, or because you have slept through the alarm, it is much better for you not to get out of bed the minute you wake up.

BODY CHECK
● As soon as you wake up stretch and yawn – enjoy it.

● Move your fingers and toes.

● Move your hands and feet in circles.

● Sit up and breathe deeply.

● Rub the palms of your hands together then press them together.

MIND CHECK
● Get in touch with your breath, become aware of its rhythm.

● Guide your breath deep down (feel it in breathing areas 1 and 2).

● When inhaling make the air flow to all parts of the body.

● Guide the flow of air by deep breathing, sighing.

● Sitting on the edge of the bed, breathe in, then slowly exhale.

While you are still in bed, start stretching your arms and legs, first under the bedclothes, then above them. Gradually stretch each part of your body, yawning as often and intensely as possible.

● **Yawning and stretching** activate your breathing, which slows during sleep. The muscles, relaxed for sleep, are "told" to get ready for the daily activities ahead.

Now wiggle your fingers and toes, or clench them or knead them. Gradually enlarge these movements so you bend the joints of your hands and feet, making circles with them to get your circulation moving.

● **The stimulated circulation** informs the heart and breath that sleeping time is over and that the rhythm of the day has begun.

Stretch your body again, breathing deeply. If you can manage a sigh or a moan as well it will send a positive spark through your mind and body.

Ease yourself upright, by gently rolling on to your side and swinging your legs on to the floor. Sit on the edge of the bed, feet on the floor, while you breathe in and out twice. Exhale and rub your hands together, inhale and keep them still with palms together.

Do this two or three times, enjoying the air flowing through your nostrils and travelling down into your body. Lightly

pressing your palms together, raise your arms to chest height, about 15 cm (6 in) from your body and breathe deeply in and out twice, turning your hands in a semicircle toward your chestbone and then out in front. Stretch yourself once more before you actually stand.

● **Your spine, muscles and** circulation are now stabilized and adjusted to the fact that your body is upright and preparing to be on the move.

A new pace

These small activities are all adjusted to the functions of your body. Slowly changing over from the rhythm of sleep to that of action changes the pace of your breath, so your mind and body are primed to start the day calmly and with assurance. It need only take five minutes to wake up well.

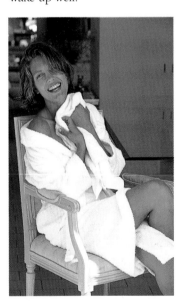

Moving into the day

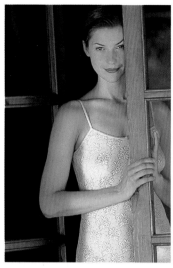

Making sure you are not in a draught, stand in front of an open window and stretch. Now make large circles with your arms, reaching high as you inhale and lowering them as you exhale. Do this a few times.

● **Your lungs are cleansed** and stale air accumulated during the night's shallow breathing will be removed.

Breathe out and roll your spine downward from head to sacrum (see p. 30), relaxing the trunk. Pause and inhale, bend your knees and roll upward, from the sacrum to the neck and head. Breathe in, lift up your arms and stretch them above your head, exhale slowly and move your arms out wide to the side, then let them hang loosely. Stand upright and enjoy breathing deeply a few times.

● **Your spine is gently** stretched as you roll it, getting rid of any local stiffness, activating the back muscles and stimulating the circulation.

BODY CHECK

● Yawn and stretch in front of an open window.

● Breathe out twice deeply while moving your arms in circles.

● Roll your spine downward, then upward, then stretch.

● Lower arms to sides, and enjoy deep, slow, effective breathing.

MIND CHECK

● With each in-breath guide the air from the sacrum along the spine.

● By the third in-breath feel your breath reach the top of your head.

● Breathe in and out twice through the nose.

● Breathe out quickly through the mouth, you'll feel the walls of the abdomen cave in and your breath in all breathing areas.

● Make sure the walls of the diaphragm cave in when you exhale.

● Feel the last calm breath moving up from your heels along the back of your legs and up the spine to the top of your head.

Energy boost

Don't just step into the shower or bath. First give yourself a massage to remove dead cells from the skin's surface and allow the pores to breathe.

● **Use a body brush (loofah),** a massage glove or even a coarse towel. The idea is not that harder is better, but you should feel happily tingly all over, with the skin vitalized, not hurt or red.

When brushing your body try to breathe out with every stroke. Start from the toes, go up the legs to your thighs, then do the hands along the arms to the shoulders. Move quickly and gently along the trunk. In the middle, brush in a circular movement over the stomach, chest and lower abdomen.

Brush all the parts of the back you can reach – with the neck start at the base of the head and move along the shoulder and right down the arm on both sides. Now you can have your shower or bath. Let your breath flow calmly under or in the warm water.

Ideally you should follow this with a short cold shower over the arms and legs, to stimulate the circulation. Rub yourself dry briskly, breathing out strongly as you do so.

Later, when you are confident of your new power of breathing, you can concentrate on letting the water dry on your skin. The morning should start with water. Half a litre (1 pint) before

BODY CHECK
● Brush your body from top to toe for two minutes.

● Have a pleasantly warm shower or bath (preferably a shower).

● Have a short cold shower over the legs and arms.

● Briskly towel yourself dry.

MIND CHECK
Mental action in this instance requires experience with breathing training because it requires hard concentration. If you can,

● Imagine your skin tingling every time you breathe out.

● In the shower guide the warmth into your hands and feet.

● As the water dries on your skin feel your breath flowing from the inside to the outside.

● When the in-breath has reached the skin's surface make your breath flow into the room like warm vapour.

Fuelling yourself

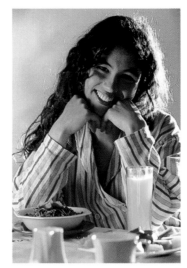

breakfast begins to restore the body's water balance. (You may not realize how much sweat and waste products your body continues to remove while you sleep). Which water you drink is up to you – from the tap, filtered or bought mineral water.
● **Your breakfast should** neither fill you up nor leave you hungry – both have a negative effect on your breathing. Herbal tea is preferable to either black tea or black coffee (if you can't do without them, weaker is better than strong). Gradually you could make the tea or coffee weaker and then substitute herbal tea. Your morning programme of waking up with breathing will make you feel much more awake and

alert for longer than coffee or tea will.

While preparing breakfast, breathe in and savour the aromas – freshly squeezed orange juice, fresh fruit, herbal tea, cereal, toast. With one finger hold one nostril closed, breathe in and smell the food, then breathe out. Do the same with the other nostril too. It will stimulate the breathing muscles and make you feel mentally awake.
● **Sit up straight while eating,** stretching your spine from the sacrum to the top of the head – the King's position in which you can clearly feel your sitting bones (see p. 42).

Before starting breakfast breathe deeply twice and eat slowly and consciously. With your mouth closed, chew in an exaggerated way so you feel the muscles are alive. Breathing in and out through the nose

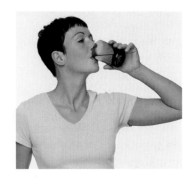

BODY CHECK
● Appreciate the smell of breakfast food and drink.

● Sit upright at the table (don't slouch).

● Move your face muscles when chewing, breathe through the nose.

● Clean your teeth with your tongue before brushing.

Last-minute tension busters

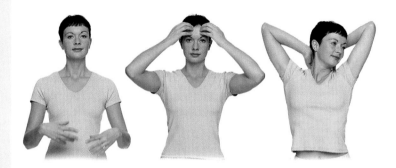

encourages blood circulation in the skin and restores vitality to the upper respiratory tract.

Before you leave the table calmly and deeply inhale and exhale once. While you are clearing dishes away clean your teeth with your tongue. This isn't a substitute for the real thing which you will do later but a way of activating the inside of the mouth and the tongue. Run the tip of your tongue along the outside of your teeth, then move it to the inside, on the upper row, then on the lower several times.

● **If you think all this activity** will extend breakfast – and you know you have little time in the mornings – don't worry. It adds only a few minutes.

Caught sight of the clock and realize it's time to run for the bus or train, grab your car keys or bicycle helmet? This is stress that is worth avoiding – here are some tips on how to do it in the minutes before you leave.

● Gently shake your hands from the wrists while breathing out, hold them still while breathing in through lips pursed as if whistling. Shape your lips as if trying to blow out a candle, exhale and send any troubling thoughts with it. Do this two or three times then resume your normal breathing.

● Curve the fingers of both hands as if holding a tennis ball. Starting at your centre forehead, tap your fingertips along your hairline down to the neck. Hum

a tune if you like. When you inhale rest your fingers and guide the flow of air in their direction. Tap fairly hard so the blood is stimulated. Do it two or three times, breathing evenly.

● Ready to go? Pause in front of a mirror, breathe in and out. Entwine your fingers together, place them behind your neck and gently lean your head back into your hands. Breathe out and pull your head up, then roll your neck down vertebra by veterbra to stretch it gently. Lift your head, give your mirror image a big confident smile and off you go into the day.

Get into the day's rhythm

Your breath during the day should flow calmly and rhythmically. It is helpful if you know the danger signs to watch for and what you can do to restore the balance.

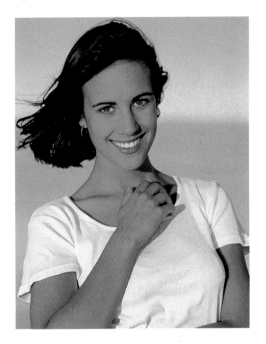

Your day can be interrupted by things that happen, like a stressful appointment, an unpleasant conversation, a sharp memo. All can influence your breathing. But there are positive things that can have an effect too – a friendly nod, a smile, an enjoyable lunch, the sound of a loved one's voice, a joke or anecdote shared. Each of these helps you breathe more deeply, giving your breath a regular rhythm and reducing its pace. When you have noted this consciously a few times, you will be able to guide your breath back to its normal rhythm ridding yourself of any panic, moods and nervousness.

Think positive

- Train yourself to become aware of positive happenings around you.
- Positive thinking deepens and stabilizes your breath.

- Watch how your breath reacts when something positive occurs. Hold on to this breathing experience as long as you can, remember its effect.

- Be the one who takes the initiative, makes the friendly gesture.
- It's easier to smile than it is to scowl.

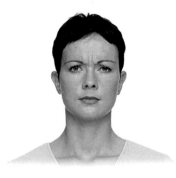

Know your negative reactions

- Become aware of how your breath reacts in situations over which you have no control.
- Work out the form it takes, its rhythm and its rate (how many times you breathe in per minute).

Dangers of holding the breath

When you stop breathing – or hold your breath – it can be because you are concentrating too hard. It can happen in an engrossing conversation or when doing something that demands your full attention; somehow you just forget to breathe! But you may also stop breathing when you are angry, when frightened or shocked, when there is a drastic change in temperature or when you experience great pain.

Whatever the cause, your breathing pattern changes and it affects other parts of the body such as the heart and blood, even the metabolism. By keeping a close eye on yourself you will soon find what makes you hold your breath. After this you can decide to avoid the situation that caused it or to train yourself to guide your breath and make it flow evenly. Turn the page for how to do this.

Guiding your breath

The most vital way to reduce stress on mind and body is to guide your breath back to its normal flow and rhythm. It is important that you recognize when your breathing pace changes and act fast – the more you practise this the quicker you will be able to attain calmness, no matter what situation you find yourself in.

To exercise and stabilize your breath, smoothing out any irregularities, follow the suggestions for reducing tension, stimulating your breathing and refinding its normal rhythm, whether you are on your own or with others.

Reduce tension

● **On your own.** Breathe out strongly three times and let your trunk and arms fall forward. When you straighten up between each out-breath, inhale as little air as possible. Breathe in while leaning forward, straighten up while exhaling. Breathe in briefly, bend forward again and breathe out all the air you can – through the mouth as in a cleansing breath.

● **In company.** Breathe out as hard as you can until you get the feeling that there is no air left in your body. Make yourself aware of this state of emptiness, then breathe in slowly. You will feel relieved.

Stimulate breathing

● **On your own.** Sit or stand and while breathing out put your hands under your armpits, then move them down the sides of your body, bending your trunk and knees until your hands reach the floor. Now inhale and guide your hands up your body, stretching your arms above your head. Exhale and move your hands down your sides again. Repeat three times.

● **In company.** Fold your arms and think of your breath entering your body, starting at the top and moving down, and leaving it by travelling from the bottom to the top. Concentrate on breathing rhythmically.

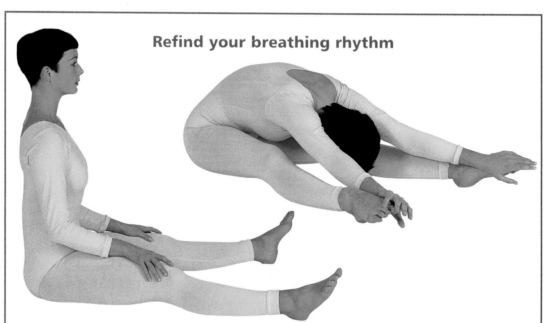

Refind your breathing rhythm

● **On your own.** Sit down with your trunk erect and forming a right angle with your thighs. Sit like this for some time without leaning back and listen to your breathing. Breathe out and let your trunk fall forward, breathe in and move back to the upright position. Swing your body as wide as possible.

● **In company.** Sit as upright as you can and concentrate on *thinking* your body is swinging. As you do so, you will find you are guiding your breathing back to its normal rhythm. Breathe out, pause, breathe in, then sigh deeply to release tension. It becomes easier with experience and the big advantage of linking your mind and breathing in this way is that people will hardly notice that you might have briefly lost your equilibrium.

Tactics to overcome shallow breathing

Shallow breathing occurs when only some of the breathing areas are used. It can happen when you're angry or afraid, nervous, under stress or simply because you've never learned to breathe any other way.

Because you take in less air when you breathe shallowly, you increase the rate of breathing to compensate and to provide enough oxygen (this is, after all, the whole purpose in breathing). The end result, however, is to put the body, and especially the heart, under stress. Shallow breathing, caused by stress, increases the stress you are under, creating a vicious circle. Here are some ways to break it.

The chest

1 Breathe in and place your hands on the wall of the diaphragm on both sides. Breathe out while applying slight pressure to your chest with your palms to make the ribs move toward the middle of the body and relax the diaphragm walls (essential if the elasticity is to be reactivated).

2 Breathe in again and allow your chest to become smaller when you exhale through the mouth. Your palms move toward the chestbone, but keep the pressure light. You should feel pleasantly relaxed. An alternative is to fold your arms across your ribcage, slightly round your back and lean forward as you exhale.

3 Repeat two or three times and breathe deeply.

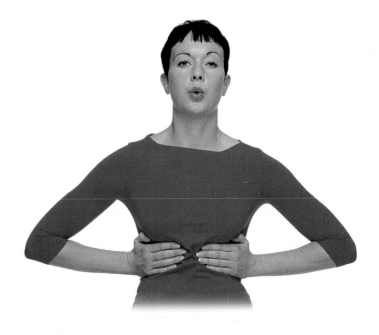

The legs

1 Cross your legs at the knee, clasping the knee on top with your nearest hand while folding your other arm behind your back. Breathe out and turn your trunk and head toward the folded arm while the knee moves in the opposite direction. You should feel a slight stretching sensation in the middle of your body. Hold the position as you breathe in and out once or twice.

2 Exhale and slowly move your trunk back to the middle, then breathe deeply. Repeat this on the other side. Finally breathe in and out through your nose.

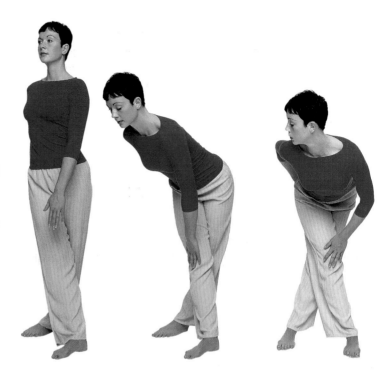

The trunk

1 Place both feet flat on the floor, hip-width apart. Rest both hands on your thighs.

2 Breathe in and bend the trunk forward, as far as you like as long as you don't feel any discomfort. Slowly exhale, moving your hands down your legs to your feet. If it's easier, rest your trunk on your thighs with knees slightly bent.

3 When you are in a comfortable position, let your arms hang loosely and stretch your neck a little. Breathe in and out three to five times, humming if you can to make the air flow slowly through the nose to the middle of the body and down into your back.

4 Make yourself aware of the movement of your breath in breathing area 1 at the back by putting your hands on the right and left side of your lumbar spine.

5 Once you can clearly feel your breath, slowly straighten up. Breathe in deeply and breathe out with a sigh. Inhale and exhale twice, then repeat the exercise.

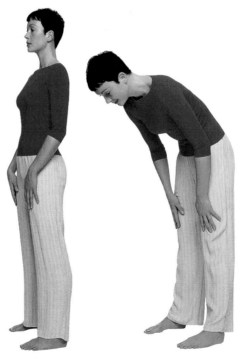

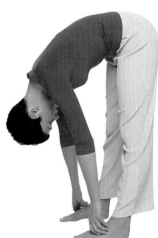

UNCONSCIOUS BREATH

Your breathing is controlled automatically by reflexes which do it all for you. But you do need to know something about this "unconscious" movement of the in- and out-breath, to know its rhythm and what may influence it. Unconscious breathing requires no apparent information or conscious thought from the brain, and the brain does not have to digest any additional information or commands. You can trust the reflexes and can simply watch and learn until you want to influence the movement consciously.

The hands

1 Put your hands together in front of you, then turn them in toward your body so your fingertips point at your chestbone and your elbows are wide.

2 Breathe out and move the fingers up along the chestbone on the central line of the body to shoulder level. Pause and breathe in through the nose.

3 As you breathe out through the nose, turn your hands to the front (describing a semicircle) so they are pointing away from you. This will calm you and deepen your breathing. Repeat steps 1 to 3 up to five times. Breathe freely and rest both hands on your thighs.

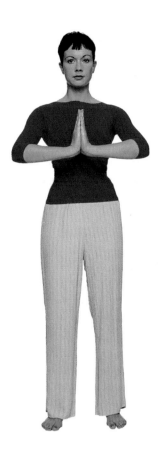

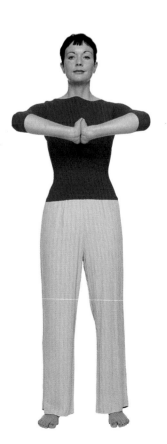

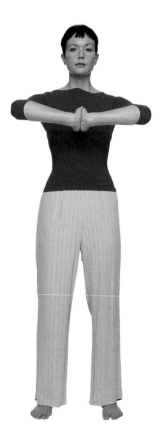

CONSCIOUS BREATH

The movement of your breath is monitored and controlled by the medulla, the brain's respiratory centre. But the breathing mechanism can also be deliberately guided and controlled. If you choose to do this you can apply the strength of your breath to greater use, ensuring that your blood is kept oxygen-rich and that all the cells of the body are kept healthy.

Letting go now and then

There are times when you have to relax to gain energy. Everything is racing around you at a speed that leaves you feeling breathless, as if the power has been turned off – and if you left it like that you would suffer.

Gain energy

When you are being affected adversely by events find time to get back to your inner self. Here are some suggestions for a "relax and gain energy" break.

● Retreat to a place where you won't be disturbed by the phone, the television or people. Sit on a chair in the King's position (see p. 25). Breathe out a few times while sighing, then breathe in deeply.

● Become aware of your breathing rhythm and guide it to the rhythm of tranquil or passive breathing. Pause after exhaling then breathe in slowly through the nose.

● Make the pause last longer. Breathe out and pause and rest while pausing – the weight of your body sinks into the chair even though you are sitting upright. This means you let go, trusting the chair to hold you. Breathe out and close your eyes, pause and open your mouth a little. This will cause your lower jaw to drop slightly. Close your mouth and take in a moderate amount of air through your nose. Breathe in and out in this way five to ten times.

● Breathe deeply, feeling the oxygen-rich air bringing your body vital new energy.

Staying alert

It may sound the opposite of the keyed-up state you would expect when alert, but when you let go and relax your concentration will automatically increase. If your concentration is low it it because you are drained of the energy you need.

● Sitting in the King's position at a table or desk, get in touch with your breath, become aware of it then breathe in and out as deeply as you can.

● Create tension in your breathing by guiding your breath deep down several times. Each time you inhale hold your breath for one or two seconds. Push your lips forward (as if blowing out a candle) and exhale through your mouth.

When you hold your breath after inhaling, you will feel your energy expanding from inside your body to all its parts. It will make you feel revitalized.

● Breathe in a few times while "sniffing" (as if you were asking "what is it that I can smell?")

When you sniff while breathing in, you gain even more energy. Imagine that the air is not only entering your body through your nose but also through your eyes.

● Once you have the feeling that you have emptied your head (no thoughts keep flashing into it) place your elbows on the table in front of you and cover your ears with your hands. Keep your shoulders relaxed and open up your chest. Now breathe in and out, and hum every time you exhale – to cause vibrations which will soon give you a clear head again.

Incidentally, you may feel that the humming sounds loud inside your head, but people around you will hardly hear it.

Resting easy

In the course of everyday life you are haunted by many different images and subjected to many demands. Sometimes there are simply too many of them and you reach the point of overload. When you're at home in the evening after that sort of day your head will be buzzing with so much information that you find it hard to relax. But you owe it to yourself to try, before it develops into excess tension which causes you to become irritable and react badly to those around you. In this state, you will have problems getting to sleep and wake up frequently during the night. Ongoing sleep deprivation can lead to stress and cause you to feel below par. This in turn makes you vulnerable to illness.

To make your day end in harmony, try any of these:

● On your way home from work, relax. Breathe out deeply and let the air leave your body in a steady flow. Be aware of the rhythm of your breath and guide it so it becomes regular.

● When you get home, allow a few minutes for yourself without diving immediately into whatever needs to be done. Find a secluded place where no one will disturb you and breathe out as you glide your palms down your trunk starting from the top. Each time you exhale move your palms a little faster – this will eventually lead to an invigorating cleansing breath. Breathe in and out rapidly a few times then give your hands a good shake

● Place your right hand on breathing area 1 at the front, the left hand on breathing area 1 at the back. Breathe in and out deeply five to seven times and become conscious of the movement of your breath between your hands. Take your hands away and breathe deeply three times.

● When you noticeably feel more relaxed, you are ready to proceed with the evening. Be conscious of keeping a tranquil breathing rhythm – this will not allow your day at work to make its way into your family or your life at home.

Getting to sleep

You need to feel relaxed and surrounded by calmness in order to get to sleep. You may have to establish a pre-sleeping habit which requires very little of you but which you enjoy. It could be a warm bath, reading a short story or a poem, browsing through a magazine that does the trick. Perhaps it is simply doing nothing at all. Going straight to bed after you've done the chores or switched off after an evening's television is not a good idea as the tension these activities cause go to bed with you, disturbing your sleep.

Your mind and body both need to be aware that you are entering a quiet phase.

● Once comfortably in bed, lying on your back, place both hands on your stomach. Each time you breathe out feel your stomach caving in under your hands, pause then imagine you are sinking into a hammock

It is important to put your thoughts to rest when entering this sleep phase, and you need to recover from one activity before engaging in another. Make your thoughts leave your body with every out-breath, just as you sent the tension out of your body. While breathing deeply keep thinking "I want to rest. I want to become calm". These constant thoughts will lull you gently to sleep.

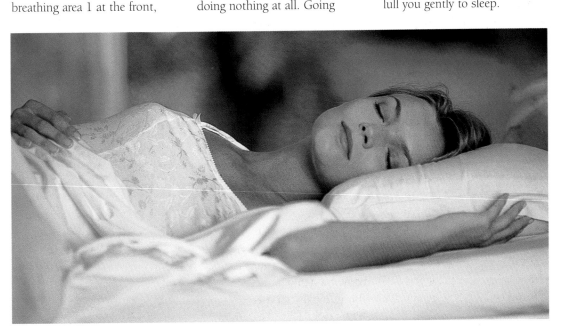

A self-help guide to everyday ailments and conditions

Yᴏu can use the breathing exercises to improve specific areas of your health. Just follow the suggested combinations to eliminate problems which affect your well-being. Do them sequentially over several days, moving on only when you have felt the benefits of the one you have completed.

Low energy levels

 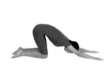 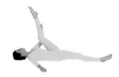

Home start: Ribs and diaphragm, 2 (p. 47)

The Cat: Stretch and strengthen, 1 and 2 (pp. 63–64)

The Cloud: Expand and accumulate, 1 and 2 (pp. 72–74)

The Root: Strength and stability, 2 and 3 (pp. 78–80)

The Ball: all (pp. 92–99)

Tiredness, chronic fatigue

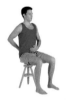 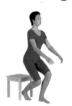 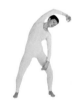 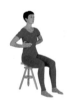

Home start: The sitting bones, 1 (p. 42)

The Pendulum: Getting into the swing, 3 (p. 50)

The Cloud: all (pp. 70–75)

The Flower: Extend and stretch, 4 (p. 90)

The Ball: Feel your breathing (p. 93), Breathe and bounce, 1 (p. 94), Tense and bounce (pp. 98–99)

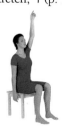

The Wave: Extend your breathing (p. 102)

Insomnia

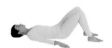

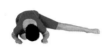

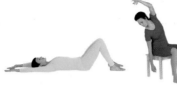

The Cradle:
Rocking and
rolling, 1 (p. 56)

The Cat: Stretch
and strengthen, 3
(p. 65)

The Flower:
Extend and
stretch, 1 and 2
(pp. 84–88)

The Wave. . . all
(pp. 100–105)

Anger, irritability

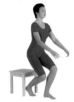

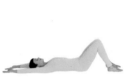

The Pendulum:
Getting into the
swing, 2 and 3
(pp. 49–51)

The Pendulum:
Regaining control
(p. 54)

The Cradle:
Rocking and
rolling, 4 (p. 61)

The Flower:
Extend and
stretch,1 and 2
(pp. 84–88)

The Wave. . . all
(pp. 100–105)

Nervous tension, stress

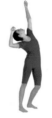

Become aware of
your breathing,
1 and 2
(pp. 38–41)

The Pendulum:
Getting into the
swing, 1 (p. 48)

The Cat: Stretch
and strengthen,
3 (p. 65) and
5 (p. 68)

The Wave:
Rhythm and
rolling (p.100)

Get out of breath when walking uphill

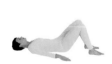

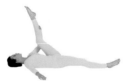

The Cradle:
Rocking and
rolling, 1 and 2
(pp. 56–58)

The Cat: Stretch
and strengthen, 3
(p. 65)

The Root.: all
(pp. 76–83)

The Ball: all
(pp. 92–99)

121

Can't breathe when swimming

 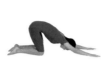

The Pendulum:
Getting into the
swing, 3 (p. 50)

The Cat: Stretch
and strengthen, 2
(p. 63)

The Flower: all
(pp. 84–91)

The Wave: all
(pp. 100–105)

Hold breath when nervous

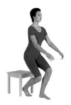 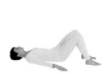

The Pendulum: all
(pp. 48–55)

The Cradle:
Rocking and
rolling, 1
(p. 56)

The Flower:
Extend and
stretch, 4
(p. 90)

The Wave:
Rhythm and
rolling (p. 100)

Throat infection

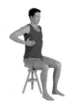 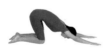 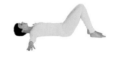

Home start: Ribs
and diaphragm,
1 (p. 46)

The Cat: Stretch
and strengthen, 1
(p. 63)

The Flower:
Extend and
stretch, 1 and 2
(pp. 84–88)

Common cold

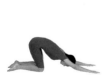

The Cat: Stretch
and strengthen, 1
and 2
(pp. 63–64)

The Cloud: all
(pp. 70–75)

The Wave:
Rhythm and
rolling
(p. 100)

The Wave:
Extend your
breathing
(p. 102)

Blocked sinuses

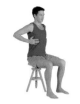

Home start: Ribs and diaphragm, 1 (p. 46)

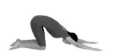

The Cat: Stretch and strengthen, 1 (p. 63)

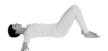

The Flower: Extend and stretch,1 (p. 84)

Stiff back

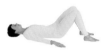

The Cradle: Rocking and rolling, 1 and 2 (pp. 56–58)

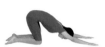

The Cat: all (pp. 62–69)

The Flower: Extend and stretch, 4 (p. 90)

The Ball: Tense and stretch (p. 96)

Slack calf muscles

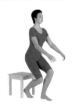

The Pendulum: Getting into the swing, 3 (p. 50)

The Cradle: Rocking and rolling, 3 and 4 (pp. 58–61)

The Cat: Stretch and strengthen, 3 (p. 65)

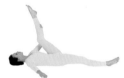

The Root: all (pp. 76–83)

The Ball: Breathe and bounce, 1 (p. 94)

Digestive problems

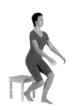

The Pendulum: Getting into the swing, 3 (p. 50)

The Cradle: Rocking and rolling, 4 (p. 61)

The Cat: Stretch and strengthen, 3 (p. 65), 4 (p. 67) and 5 (p. 68)

The Root: Strength and stability, 3 (p. 80)

The Flower: Extend and stretch, 4 (p. 90)

The Ball: Tense and stretch (p. 96)

The Ball: Tense and bounce (p. 98)

Chronic conditions

Bronchitis

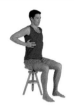 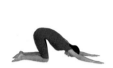

Home start: Ribs and diaphragm, 1 and 2 (pp. 46–47)

The Cat: Stretch and strengthen, 1 (p. 63)

The Cloud: all (pp. 70–75)

The Wave: Rhythm and rolling (p. 100)

Headache

 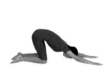 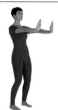 

The Pendulum: Getting into the swing, 1 (p. 48)

The Cat: Stretch and strengthen, 1 (p. 63) and 3 (p. 65)

The Cloud: Expand and accumulate, 3 (p. 74)

The Flower: Extend and stretch, 1 (p. 84)

The Wave: Rhythm and rolling (p. 100)

Low back ache

 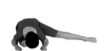

The Cradle: Rocking and rolling, 1 (p.56) and 4 (p. 61)

The Cat: Stretch and strengthen, 3 (p. 65)

The Root: Strength and stability, 4 (p. 81)

The Wave: Rhythm and rolling (p. 100)

Do...
- Take your time. Learning to use your breath well is a gradual process and you progress as you feel the benefits.
- Plan your exercise routine so you have time for it each day. The continuity of exercising helps your breathing to become instinctive.
- Be conscious of your breathing from the moment you wake.
- Be willing to learn – it stimulates your brain and makes you more alert and youthful.
- Use your breathing to give an instant energy boost or to calm yourself.
- Set yourself challenges.
- Listen to your breathing.

Don't...
- Let tiredness stand in the way of your exercise routine. Force yourself and you will feel full of vitality again.
- Breathe only through your mouth or only through your nose. To breathe well you need to do both.
- Continue to exercise if you feel discomfort. Your mind is telling you to take a break.
- Be lazy when you breathe. If you aren't using all your breathing muscles and muscle tissue. you'll feel constantly tired.
- Forget to rest between exercises. Get to know the basic positions which you can rest in easily.

Posture and breathing

Most of us spend a lot of the day sitting – to eat, to work at a desk, travel in a car, to write letters, watch television, see a play or listen to music. With each activity the seat varies and posture may suffer.

If you slump, the passage of breath through your body is hindered – and results in stress, fatigue, headaches, stomach pains, back problems and cramp in the shoulders. Such symptoms are common in workplaces where not enough attention is given to the needs of people who spend their days at a desk. Life-long spinal or muscular problems can in fact start in schools if children are forced to use inadequate furniture that is not purpose built or thoughtfully designed.

Other causes of bad posture may come from your lifestyle: carrying heavy shoulder or shopping bags which make you lopsided; too-high heels that throw the spine forward; footwear that prevents you being balanced when walking; clothing that is too tight.

Rules for good posture

From the start of the exercises you will develop a natural healthy posture which you should be able to maintain whatever type of seat you find yourself on. The aim is to take the strain off your spine.
● Sit with your trunk upright, weight resting on your pelvis. Your trunk and thighs should be at an angle of 90 degrees.
● Place your feet flat on the floor, hip-width apart, or stretch your legs out in front, keeping them parallel to each other.
● Do not cross your legs at the knees – it is bad for your circulation and restricts your breathing. Instead, if you feel it is necessary for comfort, cross your legs at the ankles, changing them over frequently.
● Keep your trunk straight and do not hollow your back. When your shoulders are relaxed, and arms by your sides, your chest will be open and you will be able to breathe freely.
● Pay attention to the position of your neck while sitting upright. Stretch it a little every so often – this will also slightly stretch your lower spine.
● Do remember, when your posture is right you should be able to feel your breath in every breathing area all day long.
● To gain the posture that's natural to you, follow the instructions for The sitting bones, 1 and 2 (pp. 42–45), then Ribs and diaphragm, 1 and 2 (pp. 46–47).

Listen to the rhythm

The breathing rhythm has three parts. The in-breath and out-breath are active. The third is passive – you pause. The pattern is: breathe out, pause, breathe in. In tranquil or passive breathing, the pace is regular, though you can slow it down or speed it up. When breathing automatically – without conscious thought – the out-breath takes longer than the in-breath which follows. When we are under stress we take longer to breathe in. Think of this when you're sitting. Alter your position and see if it affects the rhythm of your breathing.

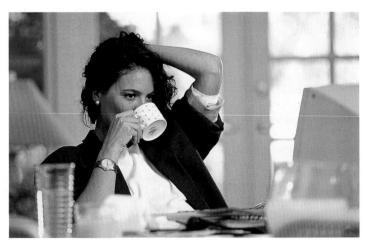

Index

A

abdomen 13, 15, 26
alertness 92–99, 118, 124
  see also concentration
anger 121
  see also irritability; temper,
  controlling
asthma 15

B

back 24, 31, 56–61, 66, 123
  disc problems 66
  low back ache 124
  see also skeleton: spine
balance 21, 23, 24, 48–55
bathing 110
blood, circulation of 7, 11, 16,
  37, 53–55, 109, 110
bones *see* skeleton
breathing 14
  abdominal 13, 15
  active 125
  areas 16–17, 22, 24, 42–47,
    70–91
  "aura" 13
  awareness 13, 38–47,
    100–105, 121
  balanced 13, 15
  bathing and 110
  breathlessness 121, 122
  bronchitis 15, 124
  chest 13, 15
  cleansing 36, 110
  colds 122
  conscious 6–9, 13, 117, 124
  contagious 13
  control and 53–55, 108, 117,
    121, 124
  daily 106–25
  deep 36, 56–61, 100–105, 109
  eating and 111–12
  energy and 62, 100, 108, 118,
    124
  exercises *see* main entry
  expanding 84–91, 100–105
  extending 102–3
  false 15
  feeling 15, 92, 93, 95
  guiding 113, 114, 117
  health and 120–25
  holding the breath 113, 122
  impulse 12, 38, 40, 41, 75, 94
  in 14–15, 36, 91, 92,
    100–105, 110, 112, 125
  lifestyle and 12, 13
  massage and 110
  mental attitude and 109, 110,
    111, 112, 113
  mouth 14, 110, 112, 124
  movement 39, 40–41, 48–55,
    68, 108
  nose 14, 36, 110, 112, 124
  out 14–15, 36, 90, 92,
    100–105, 110, 112, 125
  oxygen, wave of 100–105
  passive 125
  posture and 125
  power of 36–41
  reflex 92–99, 117
  relaxation and 118–19
  rhythm 48–55, 68, 113–14,
    117, 125
  shallow 15, 22, 115–17
  showering and 110–11
  sinuses 123
  states 90, 91
  stimulating 114
  stress 112, 113, 114, 121, 125
  swimming 122
  throat infection 122
  training 6–9, 16
  unconscious 117, 125
  waking up 108–10
  yawning 109
bronchitis 15, 124

C

cardiovascular system 11, 14, 16
chest 13, 14, 15, 115
chronic fatigue 120
circulation 7, 11, 16, 37, 53–55,
  109, 110
colds 15, 122
concentration 13, 16, 19, 27,
  108, 118
  see also alertness
confidence 7

D

daily life 106–25
depression 15
diaphragm
  exercises for 29, 46–47, 56–61,
    70–75, 92, 120, 122, 123, 125
  role of 14, 15

digestion 123
disc problems 66
dizziness, controlling 53–55
drinking 111

E

eating *see* food
emotions 22, 23
energy 24, 57, 62, 100, 108,
  118, 120
exercises 12, 13, 34–105
  abdominal wall and 26
  accumulating 72–75, 120, 124
  aim of 32
  anger, for 121
  back 24, 31, 123
  see also skeleton: spine
  balance and 21, 23, 24
  Ball 92–99, 120, 121
  bouncing 94–99, 120, 123
  breathing areas and 22, 24
  breathlessness 121, 122
  bronchitis 124
  calming 22, 53–55, 121
  Cat 62–69, 123
  chest 115
  circling 37, 109, 110
  clothing 18, 19
  Cloud 70–75, 120, 122, 124
  colds 122
  concentration and 19, 27, 33,
    118
  control, regaining 54, 121
  cooling down 27, 29
  Cradle 56–61
  diaphragm and 29, 46–47,
    56–61, 70–75, 120, 122,
    123, 124
  digestion, for 123
  effective 18–19
  effects 16, 19
  emotions and 22, 23
  energy and 24, 120
  equipment 18–19
  expanding 72–75, 120, 124
  experience 18
  extending 84–91, 120, 121,
    122, 123, 124
  feet 29, 76–83
  Flower 84–91, 122
  food and 19, 33
  hands 98–99, 117
  headache 124

health and 120–25
heels 96, 97
Home start 42–45
insomnia 121
irritability, for 121
kneeling, knees 23–24
legs 37, 76–83, 116
location 18, 33
lying 18–19, 28–29
muscles and 22, 27, 28, 29,
 32,56–75, 88, 95, 109, 110,
 123
pelvis and 20, 23, 25, 27,
 42–45
Pendulum 48–55, 122
positions 20–30
 Basic 20, 124
 Birthing 23
 Cross legged 27
 Crouching 24
 Dune 28
 King's 25, 44
 kneeling 23–24
 lying 28–29
 On all fours 24
 Package 29
 Rider's 22
 Rolling 30–31
 Seated coachman 26
 sitting 25–27
 Sphinx 23
 squatting 23
 standing 20–22
 Standing coachman 22
 Straddled legs 21
 Supine 28
 Thinking 27
 Wide hipped 21
posture and 20, 23, 102
preparation 18, 19, 32
pressure 29
quietness 19, 33
relaxation and 27, 28, 29,
 62–69, 80, 118–19
rhythm and rolling 100–105,
 121, 122, 124
ribcage and 45, 46–47, 120,
 122, 123, 124
rising 102
rocking and rolling 56–61,
 121, 122, 123, 124
rolling out tension 104–5
Root 76–83, 121, 123

routine 33, 47, 124
shaking 37
shoulders 62
side 66
sinuses 123
sitting 19, 25–27, 38–51,
 120
spine and 20, 25, 26, 28, 29,
 30–31, 56–61, 110
squatting 23
stabilising 76–83, 114, 120,
 123, 124
stamina and 22
standing 20–22
stimulating 114
strengthening 18, 63–68, 76–83,
 120, 121, 122, 123, 124
stretching 37, 63–69, 84–91,
 96–97, 98, 109, 120, 121,
 122, 123, 124
swimming 122
swinging 48–55, 120, 121,
 122, 123, 124
tapping 37
tensing 96–99, 120, 123
tension reducing 114–17, 121
throat infection 122
time 19, 33
trunk 36, 62–69, 116
twisting 66
types 18
walking 79
warming up 18, 19, 28, 31, 33,
 37, 77, 104
Wave 100–105, 121, 122
well being and 25, 28, 32, 33
yawning 109

F
fatigue, chronic 120
 see also tiredness
feet, exercises and 29, 76–83
flexibility 62–69
food 19, 33, 111–12

H
hands, exercises and 98–99,
 117
headache 124
heart 11, 14, 16, 45
heels, exercises and 96, 97
hoarseness 15
hyperactivity 18

I
insomnia see sleeping
irritability 108, 121
 see also anger; temper,
 controlling

J, K
jogging 77
joints, breathing and 16
knees, exercises and 23–24

L
laziness 15, 124
legs, exercises and 37, 76–83,
 116
leotards 18, 19
lifestyle 12, 13
lungs 11, 14, 16, 36, 45, 47,
 84–91
 see also breathing: areas

M
massage 110
medical conditions 12, 124
mobility 8, 16
mouth 14
muscles
 breathing and 16, 100,
 124
 exercises and 22, 27, 28, 29,
 32, 56–75, 88, 95, 109,
 110, 123

N
neck 125
nose 14, 36

O
organs 16, 23
oxygen see air

P
pelvis see skeleton
posture 7, 16, 83
 breathing and 125
 exercises and 20, 23, 102

R
relaxation 27, 28, 29, 62–69, 80,
 118–19
ribcage see skeleton: ribcage, ribs
running 77

S

self assessment 7, 9, 13, 18
self help 120–25
showering 110–11
sinuses 123
skeleton 42–47
  pelvis 20, 23, 25, 27, 42–45
  ribcage, ribs 45, 46–47, 86,
    120, 122, 123, 125
  shoulders 62
  sitting bones 42–47, 120, 125
  spine
    anatomy 31
    exercises and 20, 25, 26, 28,
    29, 30–31, 56–61, 87, 109,110
    rolling 30–31
sleeping 57, 108, 119, 121
stamina, exercises and 22

stomach, exercises and 95
stress 8, 15, 53, 56–61, 112,
  113–17, 121, 125
swimming 122

T

temper, controlling 53–55
  see also anger; irritability
tension see stress
thorax see chest
throat infection 122
tiredness 8, 108, 120, 124
trachea 14
training
  effects of 16
  importance of 6–9
  see also exercises
trunk, exercises and 36, 62–69,
  116

V

vertebrae see skeleton: spine
vitality see well being
voice 15

W

waking up 108–14
warming up see exercises:
  warming up
well being
  everyday 108–12
  exercises and 25, 28, 53,
    92–99

Y

yawning 109

Acknowledgments

The publishers wish to acknowledge the invaluable contribution made to this book by Laura Wickenden who took all the photographs except:

Page 8 (bottom) Robert Harding Picture Library; 9 (top) Peter Correz/Tony Stone Images; 19 J.P. Fruchet/Telegraph Colour Library; 37 David de Lossy/The Image Bank; 108 Ralf Schultheiss/ Tony Stone Images; 109 Chris Harvey/Tony Stone Images; 110 (top) The Photographers Library; 110 (bottom) Rick Rusing/Tony Stone Images; 111 (top) The Photographers Library; 111 (bottom)–113 (left) Andrew Sydenham; 113 (right) The Photographers Library; 115 Andrew Sydenham; 119 Telegraph Colour Library

Models: Annabelle Dalling, Ian Hodson, Cordelia West

Author's acknowledgments

Thank you
  Everybody who is with me on this path and gives me the confidence to develop this work
  Everybody who has helped me to write this book
  All my students and pupils who never tired of pushing me to write this book

I thank you for using this book, and knowing that we all progress each day.